Praise for *Stand Up to Stigma*

"Pernessa's book can make a difference in your life. In a powerful way, it gets to the heart of a complex issue. Many people stigmatize others without realizing it, and Seele helps readers understand what they can do to change their attitudes and actions."

—**Jeff Pegues, Justice and Homeland Security Correspondent, CBS News, and author of *Black and Blue***

"We all dream of living in a world without stigma and bias, but a quick glance at the news proves that this is a dream deferred. Pernessa Seele pulls no punches in identifying the cost of stigma and steps to take away the power of stigma and bias."

—**Rev. Dr. W. Franklyn Richardson, Chairman, Conference of National Black Churches, Inc.**

"Dr. Pernessa Seele's tireless efforts to remove disparities in health care—and wherever we need more understanding and acceptance—is nothing short of inspirational. I will gladly share this book with anyone who questions the toll that stigma takes on our human community— or the path we can take to escape it."

—**John Hope Bryant, Chairman, Operation HOPE**

"In sharing cogent reflections based upon her pioneering experiences as a courageous health advocate, Pernessa Seele squarely identifies the societal toll taken by stigma and stereotyping—and delineates the steps we can take to reaffirm the dignity we each innately possess by virtue of our humanity."

—**Natalia Kanem, MD, Acting Executive Director, United Nations Population Fund**

"Dr. Seele puts a human face on the consequences of stigma, shows the need to examine our biases, and gives me the uneasy personal reminder that as a public health official and researcher, I must drive outside my lane of numbers and statistics."

—**Willi McFarland, MD, PhD, MPH&TM, Professor of Epidemiology and Biostatistics, University of California, San Francisco, and Director, Center for Public Health Research, San Francisco Department of Public Health**

"The Balm In Gilead, founded by Dr. Pernessa Seele, has saved lives in the United States, Africa, and beyond. Through education, treatment, and prevention, Pernessa has enabled tens of thousands to walk the earth with health, hope, and wholeness. We are blessed to have Dr. Seele's narrative of healthcare and wellness in a wounded world."

—**Rev. Dr. Otis Moss Jr., international pastor, theologian, speaker, author, and activist**

Stand Up to Stigma

STAND UP
TO
STIGMA

How We Reject Fear and Shame

PERNESSA C. SEELE

Berrett–Koehler Publishers, Inc.
a BK Currents book

BERRETT-KOEHLER PUBLISHERS, INC.

1333 Broadway, Suite 1000, Oakland, CA 94612-1921

Tel: (510) 817-2277   Fax: (510) 817-2278   www.bkconnection.com

ORDERING INFORMATION

QUANTITY SALES. Special discounts are available on quantity purchases by corporations, associations, and others. For details, contact the "Special Sales Department" at the Berrett-Koehler address above.

INDIVIDUAL SALES. Berrett-Koehler publications are available through most bookstores. They can also be ordered directly from Berrett-Koehler:

Tel: (800) 929-2929; Fax: (802) 864-7626; www.bkconnection.com

ORDERS FOR COLLEGE TEXTBOOK/COURSE ADOPTION USE. Please contact Berrett-Koehler: Tel: (800) 929-2929; Fax: (802) 864-7626.

ORDERS BY U.S. TRADE BOOKSTORES AND WHOLESALERS. Please contact Ingram Publisher Services, Tel: (800) 509-4887; Fax: (800) 838-1149; E-mail: customer.service@ingrampublisherservices.com; or visit www.ingrampublisherservices.com/Ordering for details about electronic ordering.

Berrett-Koehler and the BK logo are registered trademarks of Berrett-Koehler Publishers, Inc.

PRINTED IN THE UNITED STATES OF AMERICA

Berrett-Koehler books are printed on long-lasting acid-free paper. When it is available, we choose paper that has been manufactured by environmentally responsible processes. These may include using trees grown in sustainable forests, incorporating recycled paper, minimizing chlorine in bleaching, or recycling the energy produced at the paper mill.

LIBRARY OF CONGRESS CATALOGING-IN-PUBLICATION DATA

Cataloging-in-Publication Data is available at the Library of Congress.

ISBN: 978-1-62656-937-9

FIRST EDITION

22 21 20 19 18 17   10 9 8 7 6 5 4 3 2 1

Cover design: Paula Goldstein.
Book interior production and design: VJB/Scribe.
Copyediting: John Pierce. Proofreader: Nancy Bell. Index: Theresa Duran.

This book is dedicated to *three little boys* who are growing into GREAT MEN. Each of them have moved me far away from my comfort zone in areas of stigma, fear, and shame. As I continuously watch them STAND UP to Stigma every day within their young lives, I am becoming a better human being.

I Love You Dearly!

Desmond Maurice Dease
(13 years old)

Richard Milton Smith, Jr.
(27 years old)

Darius James Dease
(41 years old)

I wish to thank Rev. Dr. Renita J. Weems for her "Just a Sister Way" love and support, which always flows freely and tells you just how it is — straight up; and to Dr. Marsha A. Martin for her friendship and lifelong commitment and dedication to end the AIDS pandemic on planet Earth. I have been truly blessed by many great individuals over the years, who answered the call to give their time and energy to The Balm In Gilead Inc. Each of them, past and present, in their own unique way, have been the wind beneath my wings and a healing balm of courage and strength.

God Is.

Blessed are they that hunger and thirst for righteousness,
for they shall be filled.

The Gospel of Matthew 5:6

—⁓—

CONTENTS

Lionel and I became dear friends in the early 1980s. I met this extraordinary, world-renown baritone through a New York City artistic magazine in which he was featured. I had just been given permission to establish the Cultural Arts Institute (CAI) within the Brooklyn Truth Center. This was a dream that I shared with my pastor at the time, The Reverend Don Nedd, who allowed me to use the space of the well-over fifteen thousand square foot church building. Over a short period of time, the CAI became a hallmark for music and dance classes, with a slate of acclaimed professional instructors. Within a few months of Lionel becoming the piano instructor, the pastor invited him to be the director of music for the Brooklyn Truth Center. With both of us living in Manhattan, we looked forward to our journey together to Brooklyn on Sunday mornings.

Over time it became very noticeable that Lionel was not well, and his condition, which he would not speak about, was worsening. All of us, including the pastor, other members, and I, became concerned about his obvious "silent" illness.

Lionel did not show up for choir rehearsal one Thursday night, and we all knew something was very wrong. A few choir members quickly decided to drive up to Harlem to Lionel's apartment to see about him. They found him slumped over in his chair. Deceased.

The pastor fully supported Lionel's mom, who arrived from Texas having just lost another son several months earlier. I also visited with his mom while she was attending to the business of her deceased son. There was never any mention of Lionel's illness or what became of his body. There was no funeral or memorial service in NYC that I knew of. Our church, however, did recognize his transition and spoke of his greatness. I can still hear my friend singing, "I Surrender All." Lionel's voice captured the writer's soul when penning that song.

Perhaps two weeks after Lionel's death, the CAI's violin teacher, another world-renown artist who lived in Harlem, called me to inquire about the cause of Lionel's death. I remained clueless.

"GRID! I bet Lionel had GRID."

I had never heard that word and remained clueless to what it meant. Gay-related immune deficiency (GRID) would become a word I would learn much about in the years to come. I will never forget the next statement Jerry made. It would be the last time we spoke. "If I got that, I would kill myself." A few weeks later, Jerry found out he had GRID, now known as AIDS, and committed suicide.

In 1989, working at Harlem Hospital, I became tormented by the lack of family and spiritual support for people who were, at that time, dying of AIDS. These were the dark days of AIDS. I was and remain baffled about the absence of compassion for people who suffer from AIDS or any disease or devastating situation in life. The results of my good intentions and neophyte understanding about HIV and AIDS was the creation of the Harlem Week of Prayer for the Healing of AIDS, which gave birth to The Balm In Gilead, now an international nongovernment organization working to strengthen the capacity of faith communities in the United States and around the globe to become a beacon of light in areas of health promotion and disease prevention — and to serve all of God's people with compassion and knowledge, not with hatred and ignorance.

This book is not about HIV and stigma. It is about the inherited social disease of stigma that continues to infect each of us in some way and is passed on continuously from one generation to the next.

I am a child of stigma, shame, and fear. I grew up a colored child with congressional rulings that mandated that I drink from most often dirty, "Colored Only" water fountains. "White Only" signs stated with cruel punishment that I could not try on any shoes or clothes in the department stores in Charleston, South Carolina. I could not walk the shores of Folly or Myrtle Beaches. In fact, I was allowed only on the colored Atlantic Beach, passing all the "white only" beaches along the 116-mile drive. My mom had to pack a big lunch for the almost three-hour drive in both directions because colored people could not eat in any of the restaurants along the way. (There were no interstate highways.) During the long ride to the beach, once a year, the bus made at least two stops near the woods so that we could relieve our bodily functions behind a tree. Coloreds were not allowed in bathrooms.

I was also an obese child. "Fatty" and "Porky Pig" were my nicknames growing up. My father was an alcoholic. I grew up living with shame and fear. Fear of the next bully, my father included, who would attack me by hitting me or calling me names or taking my personal power away just by laughing at me. Oh, and by the way, I was adopted, which really wasn't a bad thing, until I found out that everyone knew about it except me.

I have spent most of my adult years working to heal myself of my inner shame and the impact of stigma on my life. I wish I could say I am all healed. But I am not. It is a lifelong process. Throughout my career in public health and as a spiritual being who stands strong in the awesomeness of God and His omnipotent glory, I have witnessed first-hand the erroneous, messy, filth of stigma in public health and in religious communities around the world. The messy filth of stigma is certainly strong and horrific among many of my beloved Christians of all races, who often seem to hate people just as much as they love Jesus. The same can be said about many of my dear colleagues in public health. Their great intentions to save humanity from sickness and disease are equalized by their inherited, institutional, and personal biases that judge one's character, tolerance for pain, and worthiness to live by the color of a person's skin, zip code, or socioeconomic status.

Stigma is a burdensome and heavy word. It carries the weight of negative and often unfair beliefs that we hold about each other. Perhaps most tragically, stigma locks people into stereotyped boxes and denies us all the right to be our authentic and whole selves. We all have the tendency to sit on our high thrones and look low as we proclaim how progressive we've become. However, the reality is that we both perpetuate and experience the burden of stigma in our public and private lives every day.

Yet another generation of children are being taught to hate other human beings for one reason or another. When does it stop? Stigma-like bombs are intended for the destruction of lives and territories. For many of us, we have had enough. However, without purging our own realities of hate — why we hate and how we hate — we will continue to pass on to our children and their children's children the world's greatest social disease: stigma. They, too, will grow up and live out their lives in shame and fear or as unconscious bigots.

For those who agree, we must stand up to persons and institutions that choose to kill and destroy human beings on any level. We must stand up to stigma everywhere! Each of us who believes in goodness and righteousness must work to eliminate stigmas about people who are different from us. We must stand up to laws and policies that discriminate against all people. Two institutions, in my opinion, that have the greatest influence to change how we think and live together as human beings are religious and public-health institutions. Religious and public-health discrimination policies must be acknowledged and eliminated if peace and righteousness will one day inherit the earth. Stigma and discrimination, resulting in shame and fear, are powerful war tactics that play out in schoolyards, grocery stores, places of worship, Congress, and within every home, every day. Institutions are made up of people. Each of us has a responsibility to be consciously clear about each decision that is made. Is it a decision of discrimination and bias or one of peace and righteousness?

This book is about examining who we have become and why. I believe we all can stand up to stigma and change representations in our places of worship, public-health institutions, and media; we can get rid of laws and policies targeting stigmatized groups and set an example for future generations, starting with our very own children and grandchildren.

Today, with factual knowledge and my own spiritual understanding, I am a practicing Christian, and I have great respect for all of God's people who make up the diverse mosaic of religious and spiritual paths, and I am a strong advocate for public health and science.

Before launching into this work, I would like you to consider three terms. Although each term can be seen as a single, simple word, each one also carries a vast amount of meaning. What's more, these three terms are dramatically affecting our world today, and if we are to truly progress as human beings, we need to acknowledge, address, and radically alter the path they describe.

The first term I want you to consider is *civilization*, which is "the condition that exists when people have developed effective ways of organizing a society and care about art, science, etc."[1] Although the history of humanity goes back tens of thousands of years, it is only relatively recent by the historical clock that human beings have been dubbed *civilized*. Precise definitions have fluctuated over the years, but the majority agrees that being civilized refers to human societies having a high level of development in technological and cultural arenas. This is opposed to the state of being "primitive" or "belonging to or characteristic of an early stage of development."[2]

Within the context of the word *civilization* is the state of being civilized, or to be "polite, reasonable and respectful."[3] Civilized societies are cooperative by definition. It is commonly accepted by authorities that civilized humans (civilizations) first appeared around 7000–8000 BC. We are now well on our way into the twenty-first century AD. It stands to reason that if we have had nine to ten thousand years to practice and explore being civilized, then we should, today, be at a very advanced state of politeness, reasonability, and respectfulness. Unfortunately, that is not the case. In actuality, it appears that we as a civilization are regressing to a more primitive and reactionary mindset — reverting back to a period of "Dark Ages."

Take as an example the next word, *stereotype,* which is "to believe unfairly that all people or things with a particular characteristic are the same."[4] The term is more acutely defined in psychological circles as "a fixed, over generalized belief about a particular group or class of people."[5] Of course, not all stereotypes are intended to be hurtful and many are considered positive, like seeing obese people as "jolly," considering judges to be "sober," or believing that blonds "have more fun." However, it is far more common for people to focus on negative stereotypes such as Native Americans being "savage," people from Poland (Polacks) being "dimwitted," or persons living with HIV being "extremely contagious."

Stereotyping originated from a very advantageous form of behavior when civilized humanity was young. For example, judging that all cultural tribes that wore green facial paint were vicious and warlike served to prompt us to act quickly (based on previous experience of our own or those in our circle) when someone or something similar appeared to us. However, the tree of humanity, I believe, has experienced tremendous growth from its original civilized roots. Our world has exploded in technological, educational, scientific, and medical advances that cater to our civilized lifestyles. As a result of such advancements in modern civilization, we no longer have to fear such things as insufficient means of storing food, monthlong journeys on foot or horseback, or living in caves or flimsy structures. The problem is that in the midst of such advancements, the social aspect of our civilization is, at best, stagnant and, at worst, declining.

Tiya A. Miles, an American historian and professor at the University of Michigan, expounds, "Stereotypes are so powerful and resilient that they operate beyond the individual psyche to shape cultural currents and societal structures. Certain images have long operated in American culture as containers for a host of ideas that distort and belittle groups of people in ways that have material consequences."[6] Although great advances have been made over past centuries, decades, and years, stereotypical judgments about those we see or meet have become fixed in our consciousness, even if we choose not to act upon them. Stereotyping has branched into what we today call prejudice — "an unfair feeling or dislike for a person or group because of race, sex, religion, etc." — and discrimination — "the practice of unfairly treating a person or group of people differently."[7] In today's society, people are constantly favored or disfavored based on a variety of unfair judgments, many qualities of which were not chosen by them (for example, sex, ethnicity, age).

Stereotyping, prejudice, and discrimination no longer serve us as they might have many thousands of years ago. Such behaviors are now disadvantageous and work to drive

divisions between social structures that are rapidly trans-
forming into larger, united circles through globalization. As
we are witnessing, these divisions are not helpful but harmful to the advancement of civilization because of unjust,
untrue, and outright ignorant assumptions that are made
by individuals about other people. Stereotypes, prejudices,
and discriminations, therefore, serve only to disrupt the
flow of social growth specifically and cause a breakdown in
the stability of civilization in general. Thankfully, a growing
number of people are coming to an understanding about the
harmful effects of stereotyping and are moving away from
such unfounded prejudices and discriminations when making individual assessments.

This brings me to the third term, which is a lesser
known and acknowledged phenomenon that is taking place,
although it has greater potential to threaten our civilization than stereotyping, prejudice, or discrimination. This
final word is "stigma," and although related to the others, it
tends to define civilization or society as a whole compared
with the more individualistic form of stereotyping. Stigma
is defined as "a set of negative and often unfair beliefs that a
society or group of people have about something."[8] Stigmatization is broader in its effects than stereotyping because
larger numbers of people adhere to negative and unfair
beliefs. A few examples of stigma that continue to perme-
ate our humanity are those that mark all people living in the
mountains (hillbillies) as poor, white, ignorant, barefoot,
and living in shacks; all whites as dominating and prejudiced; all Muslims as terrorists; all blacks as poor and lazy;
or all Hispanics as associated with gangs that start riots and

destroy entire neighborhoods. In all likelihood, these long-standing trends of stigma are at a critical point of destroying our entire nation and way of life.

Stigma, as we all know, can involve a deliberate attempt to mark the intended victim with a feeling of lower status or shame. One might encounter a prejudiced person and never know his inner thoughts if he keeps them to himself. However, one who "stigmatizes" intends to brand the other — either by words or deeds — thereby adding to its hurtfulness as a phenomenon.

To our shame as human beings, we are witnessing the negative results of our ever-festering stigmas, which are rising to an uncomfortable and dangerous regularity throughout the world. We are witnessing it in the United States, which is considered to be one of the most civilized nations on earth. We are witnessing it in Europe, which has centuries of experience more than the United States in civilizing its peoples. We are witnessing it in Russia, China, Australia, and practically every other country. Various groups, cultures, religions, media outlets, and even governments are busy fanning the flames of stigma, which have risen to feverish and destructive levels of assault on nations of people. Perhaps what we are witnessing is the result of our ignoring the stronghold of stigma that has festered for generations against individuals and groups of people. Perhaps it is due to the rapidity of globalization, merging together peoples from various religious, ethnic, linguistic, or other backgrounds. Regardless, these are not excusable reasons. However, if we are to progress as civilized human beings, we must quell the rise of stigma by actively addressing the issues, educating the masses, and coming together as one kind . . . humans.

This book addresses the ever-present and perpetual sting of stigma, how stereotypes develop, the processes and effects of stigma, the levels of intervention that are needed, the need and process to change cultural thinking regarding this subject, and practical ways that stigma can be managed to create a healthier and more fulfilling environment for all.

CHAPTER 1

The Venom of Stigma

Stigma is a simple, two-syllable word. Yet because of an array of sociological factors, for many people it creates powerful impressions and emotions that always conjure up a variety of uncomfortable and even hurtful feelings. Many people may not be familiar with the term *stigma*, while others may refer to it only on a casual basis. Still others believe that the very injustices that the word represents have long been removed, or at least drastically reduced, in our "civilized" culture. However, is that really the case? No! It is not! For too many people in our society, we wear the impact of stigma like flaky, dry skin. The continuous application of lotion to cover up the unappealing, flaky, dry cells is a perpetual, daily exercise that almost never eliminates the problem. The human skin is our largest organ. It consists of three layers and is made up of mesodermal tissues that adapt to the internal and external environmental conditions of our bodies to protect our inner muscles, skeleton, and other organs. Our top layer of skin, often dry, flaky, and wrinkled, depending on our age, is called the stratum corneum. Its primary function is to protect us from the environmental conditions of the earth — or society, community, or family in the case of stigma.

Everyone experiences stigma at some point in their lives. Being the recipient of stigma is painful, regardless of the situation. However, becoming stigmatized because one brings a peanut butter and jelly sandwich to elementary school every day cannot begin to compare with the daily encounters of stigma experienced by millions of people as the result of culture and inherent systems of mass hatred of fellow human beings — systems that have been bred into existence through intergenerational words, thoughts, actions, and policies.

During these early years of the twenty-first century, we are witnessing the severe impact of ingrained hatred of populations in a civilized society. Among many persons presently living on planet Earth, there is a longing for the continuation of stigma and fear through legislative polices that will reconstruct or keep systems in place that render people fearful, hateful, and helpless for many generations to come. At the same time, there is hope and protest among others who want to dismantle stigma and hate of every kind and on every level, resulting in the birth of the next generation of human beings living in peace among themselves and within themselves.

Stigma is a devastating social disease in our world. The coherent progression of hate, fear, and shame for centuries has widely spread this infectious, debilitating social disease. Stigma kills millions of human beings of all ages, races, and creeds every day.

As with all diseases, it is important to first find the root cause. Is the disease caused by a bacteria, virus, or parasite? How is it transmitted — perhaps like malaria, a virus carried to human beings by female mosquitoes of the genus *Anopheles*? Or is stigma transmitted between two human beings when they encounter each other's body fluids — such as blood — when one person's blood is infected with the virus? This would suggest the continuous transmission of the virus and the disease, as is the case of the human immunodeficiency virus (HIV) that causes AIDS.

The first step in understanding the terms that define and affect society and all human beings that make up our world is to go to the roots of those terms. If you trace the root meaning of the volatile word *stigma,* you will find that it originates from the Greek language and culture. In the world of the ancient Greeks, those who were considered "lesser than" — such as criminals, traitors, the mentally ill, and slaves — received a mark (stigma) that was burned, cut, or branded into their skin. This visible mark announced that these human beings were blemished, defective, or otherwise outcast and should therefore be shunned and avoided by the general public.

Initially I called this chapter "The Sting of Stigma." However, a sting is usually considered a quick, sharp pain that oftentimes contains poison. There are so many over-the-counter antibiotics for a mere sting that I felt the word misrepresented the extreme violence and lasting effects of stigma on individuals, populations, and the communities to which they belong. On the other hand, *venom* conjures up in my mind the most terrifying predators in the world — snakes and scorpions. I personally have an extreme aversion to snakes (all kinds) and scorpions, viewing them with a hatred so strong and an almost toxic anger that I just have a desire to kill them. I know these animals don't deserve to be judged so harshly, but their cultural baggage is hard to avoid. The effects of stigma in our world, both historic and present, are the result of conscious poisoning with an undeniable desire to kill the mind, body, and spirit of another human being.

It is well documented that in the United States, there is a longstanding history of stigmatizing people who are deemed different. The Pilgrims who arrived in 1620 were escaping governmental and religious persecution. Ironically, the Puritans who followed in 1630 identified religious lawbreakers with bright letters that were worn on their clothing or by letters burned into their chests, including A for adultery, D for drunkenness, and B for blasphemy.[1] These Reformed Protestants sought to "purify" anything and anyone that did not meet their definition of the world as they saw it through their scriptural interpretation of the Bible. Criminals, "savage" Native Americans, African slaves, migrants, women, and others who were deemed offenders of ordinances and laws or who were simply different were often branded, disfigured, or otherwise marked in some fashion for identification, punishment, and lifelong shaming.[2]

We in the United States no longer impose the barbaric practice of physical disfiguration or marking as a means to identify certain categories of people, but we must grapple with the reality that almost four hundred years after the arrival of the Pilgrims, the interwoven fabric of stigma and its impact are on full display. The long-lasting protocol of applying stigmas to people or groups that we think deviate from what is normal remains an effective, behavioral intervention. The marks may no longer be physical brands, but the damage is most definitely etched into the psyche, which can often manifest in physical illness or death. History is filled with examples of past atrocities of stigmatism that not only stained our country but set the foundation for the sustained culture of stigma, hate, and fear in which we are all continuing to live.

Stigma against Native Americans

The effects of the US genocide on Native Americans are not readily talked about within the borders of the United States or on the world stage. The scope of the history, values, and contributions of Native people that is taught in American classrooms is extremely limited, at best. To give even the smallest sense of the stigma placed on "first peoples," consider how easy it is to complete this sentence: "The only good Indian is a . . . " Atrocities committed against Native Americans by European settlers and the established United States government have been extreme. A few of us might argue that the extremes continue. It is estimated that more than ten million Native Americans occupied the territory now known as the United States when European explorers first arrived. However, by 1930, the US census counted 332,000 Native Americans and 334,000 in 1940.[3] The sheer numbers involved in this decimation can be considered as nothing less than a real attempt at genocide, yet the US government remains silent, by and large, while chastising other nations for similar acts.

As the people of the young United States spread west across the continent, Native Americans were increasingly found to be occupying land that was considered valuable for farming, mining, logging, traveling, and the like. Native American tribes were systematically eliminated by force through starvation (destruction of crops and depletion of wildlife), exposure (causing members to flee during harsh weather), poisoning of food and water sources, disease (trading disease-infested items), and the outright slaughter of entire encampments (men, women, children, and elderly). More than five hundred treaties were made between the US government and Native Americans, but the majority of those (if not all) were changed, broken, or nullified when the interests of the government and/or corporations required it.[4] Many of these "Indian treaties" are still in existence and enforced today, although they are greatly reduced in their effectiveness.

Today, according to the 2010 US census, there are only 2.5 million Native Americans (inclusive of American Indians and Alaskan Natives), with about one million living on reservations.[5] Most Native Americans living on reservations do so in extreme poverty and squalor. The mental and physical health of reservation Natives are far worse than that of the general American public. Tuberculosis is 600 percent higher, diabetes is 189 percent higher, alcoholism is 510 percent higher, and suicide is 62 percent higher, and of Native Americans over twelve years of age, one out of ten becomes a victim of a violent crime every year.[6] Although conditions have been slowly improving over recent years, many Native Americans, especially the younger generations, are choosing to leave their tribal communities to pursue higher education and a better life in mainstream society. However, they have to continuously overcome hurdles of discrimination from peers, schools, housing authorities, health-care providers, businesses, and other segments of our society that still consider them to be lesser beings.

The reality is that mainstream society continues to be disrespectful and intolerant of Native people. The present fight of the Standing Rock Sioux Tribe, which began in 2016 against the Dakota Access Pipeline, is evidence of the continual disrespect of culture, land ownership, and tribal traditions that Native people still endure.[7] The Standing Rock Sioux Tribe, once a part of the Great Sioux Nation, is fighting to stop the construction of a pipeline that would, when linked with other pipelines, carry 470,000 barrels of oil per day from western North Dakota to Illinois.[8] After the pipeline was deemed too risky to be constructed near Bismarck, the capital of North Dakota, because of the possibilities of contaminating the water supply, it was rerouted to run parallel to the Standing Rock Sioux reservation, under Lake Oahe and the Missouri River, which borders the reservation.[9] The Standing Rock Sioux Tribe, like the people of Bismarck, is concerned about the possibilities of major environmental disasters, such as oil spills and water contamination, as well as the cultural threats that are being cast upon them. According to Standing Rock chairman Dave Archambault II, in his address to the Human Rights Council of the United Nations in Geneva, this action is yet another US violation of an existing Indian treaty.[10] It's noteworthy that the Obama administration halted both the Dakota Access

Pipeline and the Keystone XL Pipeline, citing safety and America's commitment to fighting climate change.[11] The Keystone XL Pipeline is a $7 billion project of TransCanada, which is constructing this oil vessel from Alberta, Canada, to Nebraska. It will at some time in the future connect with an already existing oil pipeline that runs from Oklahoma to the Gulf Coast.[12] Within five days of taking office, newly elected President Donald Trump — who boldly called Massachusetts Senator Elizabeth Warren "Pocahontas," without hesitating to disrespect her Native American ancestry, the direct family descendants of Amonute (known to us as Pocahontas), and all Native people — signed an executive order reauthorizing the completion of both the Dakota Access Pipeline and the Keystone XL pipeline along with the removal of thousands of protestors who were camped near Lake Oahe.[13]

Images of Native people as savage and unworthy of land as well as of life are being witnessed every day in our twenty-first century mainstream society. When we think of Native people, we most likely bring forth images of red-skinned men in enormous headdress costumes or savages riding on horses killing white men, women, and children. *New York Times* reporter Jack Healy, in an article published September 13, 2016, provides a glimpse of the present-day cultural divide and racial attitudes toward Native people regarding the pipeline. In the midst of only peaceful protests and demonstrations, Bruce Strinden, the commissioner of Morton County, North Dakota, and also a part-time rancher, shared in an interview the unwarranted historical fears and attitudes of surrounding white residents. He stated, "These ranchers, it's their livelihood. If somebody would come and set fire to their hay reserves and come and cut their fences and cause their livestock to get loose, that causes real problems."[14] On the other side, Jana Gipp, a member of the Standing Rock Sioux Tribe, who was also interviewed, stated that most people "don't know that we're hard workers. We don't all drink. We have jobs. We have to support our families."[15]

Stigma against African Americans

There are many historians, scholars, and individuals who try to deny the truth, but the lasting and present-day stigma of racism in America is the direct effect of the US holocaust of Native Americans and the American slave trade, which was used in the colonies between 1607 and 1776 and then flourished for almost another one hundred years. African men, women, and children were sold, bought, and bred for the purpose of the machine of slavery, which was essential to the economic empire of the South. From the early 1700s to the Civil War, enslaved people outnumbered free whites in places like South Carolina. Slave ownership meant an individual was legal property and could be separated from family members at the will of his or her master. During slavery, black people were "marked" for ownership, and offenses such as disobedience, insubordination, running away, poor work, and others were normally met with fierce reprisals, including, but not limited to, whipping, cutting off body parts, branding, and deprivation of food and shelter. Rape and physical abuse by white men were common practices against black slave women and men.

Although the ratification of the thirteenth amendment on December 6, 1865, ended slavery, Americans, both black and white, suffer from a condition that has been termed *post-traumatic slave syndrome*. Dr. Joy DeGruy, sociologist, researcher, educator, and author, outlines this theory in her book, *Post Traumatic Slave Syndrome*, which explains that necessary, adaptive survival behaviors that black people gained through multiple generations of living in a traumatic society where social norms and culture framed black people as "inherently and genetically inferior to whites" are now embedded in the psychic consciousness of black Americans. Dr. DeGruy suggests that these multigenerational, maladaptive behaviors of African Americans are the results of systematic and structural racism and oppression, which includes lynching, Jim Crow laws, and mass incarceration.[16]

I contend that white Americans are also suffering from post-traumatic slavery syndrome. What else would cause Dylann Roof, a twenty-one-year-old white man from Eastover, South Carolina, to travel to Charleston (102 miles from his home) to attend a Bible study class led by the pastor of Emanuel African Methodist Episcopal Church and then open fire, killing nine of the attending parishioners, including the pastor? In 2015, website evidence and Roof's own reasoning for the mass killing were that he wanted to start a race war in America.[17] Emmanuel AME Church was established as an extension of the Free African Society led by Bishop Richard Allen, founder of the African Methodist

Episcopal Church (AME) in 1787.[18] The church has a long history of leading social injustice movements in the South. Truly, racism in America is America's longest war.

The teachings of white supremacy, the perpetual learned behavior of hatred toward black people, and the continuous existence of the Ku Klux Klan and other hate groups entwined in American culture are evident in the present-day effects of slavery on our society. They are the direct impact of post-traumatic slavery syndrome on white America. Many blacks have shattered the glass ceiling of success. However, the current political climate and realities, which include far too many police killings of unarmed African Americans, provide daily evidence that regardless of class or economic status, African Americans are far too often singled out for unfair treatment. However, long is the list of stories with discriminatory themes that tell of the pursuit of blacks to live the American dream. One of the richest women in the world, Oprah Winfrey, has shared her stories of being discriminated against when attempting to purchase items in exclusive high-end stores when her identity was not yet known or recognized. Surely, I could write another book about my very own stories of discrimination when growing up in the segregated South and living in the North during six decades of my life thus far.

The continuous stereotyping of blacks as lazy, uneducated, violent, unfit, and unclean throughout three centuries in the United States has resulted in hatred and stigma that continue to lead to job denial and unemployment, mass criminal conviction and incarceration, poor health-care services, inadequate housing conditions, inferior educational opportunities, denial of basic rights, and much more. Outright slavery may have been officially abolished, but slave-like conditions and treatment clearly continue to plague black communities across the country. For example, the War on Drugs (1971 to present) has overly targeted blacks, resulting in skyrocketing incarceration numbers. According to Michelle Alexander, who has helped to expose the problem, there are more "black men in prison or jail, on probation or parole than were enslaved in 1850, before the Civil War began."[19] That is a sobering statement that reveals that the enslavement of black men has not ceased but shifted from the slave master's fields to imprisonment and close monitoring. According to the November 2011 *Archives of General Psychiatry*,[20] black and Asian adolescents ages twelve to seventeen are much less likely to turn to drugs or alcohol, whereas Native American and white teens have the highest rates of drug abuse in our nation today.

Interestingly, as the nation begins to focus on drug addiction among white suburban youth, solutions are focused on legislative appropriations for drug rehabilitation programs and not incarceration for petty drug possession. Drug addiction is a public-health crisis in our country. However, the primary intervention for this public-health crisis among thousands of black men and women for the past fifty years has been jail sentences resulting in felonies that legally revoke all voting-rights privileges for one's entire lifetime.

There are volumes of examples of inhumane treatment of African Americans within the health-care industry that are sickening and appalling. African Americans were both pleased and, quite frankly, disappointed that it took so long for a US president to apologize for any one of the horrendous health-care injustices inflicted upon black people over the past centuries. This occurred when then-President Bill Clinton, on May 16, 1997, issued a formal apology for the Tuskegee Study of Untreated Syphilis in the Negro Male.[21] This appalling experiment conducted by the US Public Health Service is documented as the "longest nontherapeutic experiment on human beings" in the history of medicine and public health. The lingering effect of the Tuskegee Syphilis Study and so many other documented atrocities is very evident in the alarming rates of health disparities among African Americans and in their distrust of the health-care industry in the United States.

After a mission trip to the United States in January 2016, the United Nations' Working Group of Experts on People of African Descent concluded that the history of slavery in the United States justifies reparations for African Americans. This working group is composed of human rights lawyers from around the world. Their findings were presented to the United Nations Human Rights Council on Monday, September 25, 2016, in Geneva, Switzerland. The working group report includes the following statement:

> In particular, the legacy of colonial history, enslavement, racial subordination and segregation, racial terrorism and racial inequality in the United States remains a serious challenge, as there has been no real

commitment to reparations and to truth and reconciliation for people of African descent. Contemporary police killings and the trauma that they create are reminiscent of the past racial terror of lynching.[22]

Sadly, in these uncertain days of President Donald J. Trump and the increase of racial violence in the United States, the sustained hatred of black people and the commitment to return to the days of slavery (Make America Great Again) do not allow for much political movement in the direction of reparation as recommended by the UN Working Group of Experts on People of African Descent. Further, James Porter, National Rifle Association president, during his speech to the NRA's reported 4.5 million members, called President Barack Obama a "fake president," Attorney General Eric Holder "rabidly un-American," and the US Civil War the "War of Northern Aggression." He further repeated his call for training every US citizen on how to use military firearms so that each person would be allowed to defend themselves against tyranny.[23]

CHAPTER 2

The Audacity of Stigma

The venom of stigma is never solely directed at one population. Poison spreads. Rooted in the fabric of American history, many groups of migrants have been assaulted by stigma from those who came to American shores before them. The first migrants, the Pilgrims, dismantled the nations of Native Americans and brought African men, women, and children to these shores as slaves, thus giving birth to centuries of framing hatred for human beings for one reason or the other — especially a person's skin color, which, among descendants of slaves or Native Americans, is a common theme of stigma in America. However, immigrants from Italy, Poland, Ireland, Russia, and Asia in the early 1900s all experienced America's wrath of stigma.

Today, it is "undocumented immigrants." Over eleven million people have found home in America for one reason or another over the years. These eleven million human beings are from every region of our world and are being deported in masses. America has always been a refuge for those who seek a better life and for those who seek safety from inhumane treatment or danger. Unfortunately, the actions of our current political leaders appear to be closing our doors of refuge. The political action behind "Make America Great Again" may include experimenting with "ethnic and religious cleansing in America" through mass deportation of undocumented immigrants and revoking thousands of visas for those who desire to embrace the statement found on the Statue of Liberty, still standing in New York City's harbor since her dedication in 1886. She still holds her torch of freedom.

Give me your tired, your poor,
your huddled masses yearning to breathe free,
The wretched refuse of your teeming shore.
Send these, the homeless, tempest-tossed to me,
I lift my lamp beside the golden door!"

Since the forty-fifth president of the United States took office, Muslims and Jews have been experiencing unprecedented attacks in the United States. After less than one hundred days of Trump being in office, the Jewish and Muslim communities have seen an increase in the number of their synagogues or mosques being burned or defiled. In addition, several Jewish historical cemeteries in various cities have been desecrated. One must ask the question: Will it ever end?

One of the most noted times in recent history occurred in Nazi-ruled Germany prior to and during World War II, when individuals considered to be "less than" were not only marked but burned alive. The desire to rid the country (and ultimately the world) of people considered to be inferior to the German race led to unimaginable atrocities against them. History has focused on those with a Jewish background as being the sole target of such stigmatism, and indeed they were the group most persecuted. However, more than five million non-Jewish persons were also singled out and demonized by the Nazis.[1] These other groups included Catholic priests, Jehovah's Witnesses, homosexuals, gypsies, anarchists, communists, and those with physical and mental disabilities. In many cases, an intricate system of badges stitched onto clothing or worn as armbands was used to identify various groups, but permanently tattooing numbers and various marks onto the flesh was a widespread practice as well. In 1939, at the beginning of World War II, Jewish refugees were denied entry into the United States because, according President Franklin Roosevelt, they posed a serious threat to national security.[2] Today, seventy-eight years later, President Trump, in the name of national security, is using his executive power to block the entry of thousands of refugees from war-torn countries who are seeking refuge in the United States. History is a witness that the stigma placed upon Jewish people is alive in the twenty-first century. We can only hope and pray that as we move through this century, more and more human beings will stand up and end stigma.

Stigma against Asians

As early as the 1800s, both Chinese and Japanese people were encouraged to migrate to the United States because they were seen as a source of cheap labor needed to build our rapidly expanding nation. However, because many were carriers of yellow fever, Asians were quickly dubbed with the stigma "Yellow Peril," and immigration from China was halted completely by the 1882 Chinese Exclusion Act.

Japanese laborers were then targeted to fill company slots, which rapidly increased their population. Many Japanese citizens quickly moved from base workers to owners of homes, small businesses, and farms. This led to discriminatory laws being passed that denied the Japanese from gaining citizenship, owning land, or even marrying outside their race. In many areas throughout the country, the Japanese were further denied home purchases, certain jobs, and access to unsegregated schools.[3] The Immigration Act of 1924 finally placed an immigration ban on anyone from East Asia.

Anti-Japanese sentiment remained strong up to World War II, especially in California. When Japan attacked Pearl Harbor, the underlying stigma erupted into outright persecution of Japanese American people and communities. Harsh treatment of prisoners by the Japanese military, together with overly stigmatized propaganda from US media sources, created an image in the American psyche that the Japanese were subhuman or even animals. The result was that as many as 120,000 Japanese citizens and migrants were rounded up and held in internment camps until the end of the war.[4]

Japanese American and AIDS activist Suzi Port, who is widely known for her pioneering work in providing services for people with HIV and AIDS in New York City in the early 1980s, lived in Harlem at a time when Japanese American doctors were not allowed to deliver babies in any hospital south of 125th Street. Suzi, now eighty-one years old, was born in Harlem Hospital. Women giving birth to Japanese American babies between 1930 and 1960 — were allowed only in all-segregated hospitals. Suzi's bold stories about her Hawaiian-born father and her immigrant mother from Japan are those of terror and sorrow. Because she was born in Japan, Suzi's mother was put under house arrest during World War II. She wasn't allowed to go more than two miles from her house without checking with the FBI. As a child, Suzi had no knowledge why her mother kept the shades drawn on the windows or why her mother did not attend major events that were so very important to her and her sister growing up in New York City. Now, in a time when Suzi is supposed to be enjoying retirement and reflecting back on the joys of her life, the horrors of being a Japanese American in New York City during World War II are lasting scars on her heart.

Today, Mexican Americans and Muslim Americans are at the center of America's wrath of stigma. One thing is for sure in America: learning from our mistakes does not come easy — if it ever comes at all.

Stigma against Women

Certainly, we cannot close this chapter without talking about discrimination and stigma against women.

Hillary Clinton in 2016 became the first woman in the United States to be the presidential nominee of a major political party. This great moment in history came ninety-six years after the nineteenth amendment to the US Constitution, which gave women the right to vote. As the first female elected to the US Senate from the state of New York, Hillary Clinton was one of only twenty women to hold one of the one hundred seats in the Senate. Of the 535 Congressional seats, women fill only 18 percent, and of the governor positions across our nation, women hold that office in only five of the fifty states.[5] In her first interview after her devastating defeat to Donald Trump, with Nicholas Kristof of the *New York Times,* Mrs. Clinton spoke about the reality of accepting the fact that misogyny played a role in her loss. In his reporting, Mr. Kristof expounded on Mrs. Clinton's frank conversation:

> She noted the abundant social science research that when men are ambitious and successful, they may be perceived as more likable. In contrast, for women in traditionally male fields, it's a trade-off: the more successful or ambitious a woman is, the less likable she becomes (that's also true of how women perceive women). It's not so much that people consciously oppose powerful women; it's an unconscious bias.[6]

It wasn't so very long ago that women were forced to take lowly, demeaning positions (hawkers [street sellers], cleaners, bakers, seamstresses, prostitutes) in the workforce (if they were able to work at all) and were forbidden to vote, hold positions of authority, sign contracts, or own property.

Still today in the United States, women, black women in particular, have to constantly deal with the stigma of being weaker, less intelligent, less able to lead, more distracted, and so on. It is often heralded in American society that women have obtained equality with men, but the facts fail to support that claim.

Just ask the 2015 World Cup soccer champions, the US Women's National Team, whether America recognizes women as equal to men. Members of the team have filed a complaint with the Equal Employment Opportunity Commission claiming that the women's team should be paid the same amount as the US Men's National Team, which actually finished eleventh in the World Cup competition in 2014. According to the complaint, members of the US Women's National Team are paid between 28 and 62 percent less than the men, depending on the kind of match. Against a top opponent, each man earns as much as $17,625 for an exhibition match and is paid no less than $5,000 even if the team loses. However, even if they win every game, the women are paid a maximum of $4,950 each. And the women are paid only for the first twenty exhibition games they play each year, which is grossly unjustified. That's it. Men get paid for each game, no matter how many exhibition games they play. The men's team earned $9 million in the 2014 World Cup for losing in the sixteenth round, while the women's team made $2 million when they won the 2015 World Cup Championship.[7]

In honoring her dear friend Lorraine Hansberry, author of *A Raisin in the Sun*, Nina Simone, in 1969, penned words that ignited a flame within little black girls like me growing up in the land of Jim Crow. However, it would not be until Sista Aretha Franklin sat down at the piano and vocally preached did "To Be Young, Gifted and Black" become a blazing fire in my soul. "When you feel really low / Yeah, there's a great truth you should know / When you're young, gifted and black / Your soul's intact." As a child, I could not imagine that a new dimension would need to be added to the struggle in my years ahead — To Be Young, Gifted, Black and a Woman!

Black women have suffered long through exploitation and persecution at the hands of outside forces and also within our families or those very close to us. My Uncle Otis, whom I loved and adored, was a school principal and gate-keeper of our family. Back in the day when I was a colored child in Lincolnville, South Carolina, a black man who had risen to the level of principal was revered as a community giant, not to mention the godly status he held within the family. Uncle Otis had the last word in our family on the career choices or dreams of all up-and-coming adults. I often wonder what would have become of my first cousin, who dreamed of becoming a journalist. Her career choice was slashed by my uncle, who declared that both her black skin and her gender rendered it impossible for her to seek a career in journalism. I believe the trajectory of my uncle's limited vision of what this young woman could become because of her gender and race thumbtacked my cousin's life with many, many years of internal stigma, fear, and self-doubt.

For the record, ten years later, when it was my time to declare my path, I defied my uncle's disapproval and attended an out-of-state school in Atlanta. With his authoritarian rule, he declared to my mother, his baby sister — who, like him, had obtained a college degree (they were only two of eleven siblings who went to college) — that I must attend one of the two historical black colleges in Orangeburg,

South Carolina. Further, I was to live off campus with him and his family. Standing up to my uncle (with the support of my mother), I followed my dream and attended the college of my choice. The lessons I learned at Clark College, now Clark Atlanta University, prepared me for the world in which I continue to live — and I am still Young, Gifted, Black and Woman!

Most of my career life has been spent mounting an attack from the trenches of the war zone of HIV and AIDS. Fighting a virus that knows no boundaries is very hard. At the same time, also fighting racial and gender bias on the battlefield is sickening, at best. A lot can be said about the biased limitations and lack of respect placed on a black woman–led organization by both white and black gay and heterosexual men. However, the more important story is the limited resources and attention black women living with HIV have received over the years. In 2014, four times as many black women were diagnosed with HIV than were Hispanic women, and 3.5 times as many than white women. Sixty-five percent of all new HIV/AIDS cases are among African American women, who represent a broad spectrum of socioeconomic backgrounds.[8] Yet, only limited resources are targeted to preventing HIV among women or caring for them. Factors that increase the risk of black women getting HIV include having relationships with black men released from prison, stigma, poverty, and the negative perceptions about people with HIV in black communities. Also contributing to the high risk of HIV among African Americans are decisions to hide their high-risk behaviors or conditions, which are influenced by stigma, fear, shame, discrimination, and negative perceptions about being HIV positive.

One of my colleagues in the HIV movement, and truly a hero in my book, is Dázon Dixon Diallo, founder/executive director of SisterLove. Sister Dázon's life commitment to struggle for women's human rights and reproductive justice has established SisterLove as an international movement with a mission "to eradicate the impact of HIV and sexual and reproductive oppressions upon all women and their communities in the US and around the world." Because I do not speak with Dázon often, she probably does not know how much I admire her work and the extraordinary gifts of her soul. One of so many stories about women across the globe touched and saved by SisterLove is of Phyllis Malone, an Atlanta resident. Ms. Malone shares her story in "Everyone Has a Story," a video training series produced by SisterLove to empower black women who are HIV positive to share their stories and manage their condition. During her interview with Rod McCullom, Ms. Malone stated, "I was diagnosed in 1996. I went to jail and was in prison . . . When I was released, SisterLove gave me transitional housing and later helped me find a house! I stopped taking my meds for about two years. But I returned to SisterLove. I don't want to forget my story. My past made me who I am today."[9]

Needless to say, women are far better off than one hundred, two hundred, or more years ago. We can vote, own property, and sign contracts, and we have more opportunities to acquire quality education, obtain top job positions, and hold public leadership seats. Although conditions for women have improved greatly, there are still concerning issues about suppressed educational opportunities, unequal pay, and greater hurdles to achieving high corporate and government positions. Some statistical examples are as follows:

EDUCATION

When it comes to out-of-school suspensions, African American girls placed the highest in the nation over the 2011–12 school year at 12 percent.[10] In comparison, only 2 percent of white girls received the same punishment during the same period.

EMPLOYMENT

Women make up two-thirds of those making the federal minimum wage or less (tip-based jobs).[11] Women of color make up 22 percent of minimum-wage workers.

Women make up almost half the US workforce, yet they typically make only seventy-eight cents against every dollar made by white males. The condition is worse for Latina women, who pull in only fifty-four cents against each dollar.

Obviously, there is still a lot of work to do in order for women to reach that coveted position of equality.

The Empire of Shackles

All of us have the tendency in this day and age to "sit high and low" while proclaiming how progressive and civilized we've become. However, the reality is that we experience the burden of stigma in the United States in both our public and private lives every day. If we are honest with ourselves, it becomes clear that we often "mark" people in our society, especially if they are people of different color or ethnicity. Either openly or privately, we stigmatize those people who have been incarcerated, are drug addicts, live in low-income neighborhoods, are lesbian or gay, have debilitating disabilities or diseases (such as HIV, cancer, or cerebral palsy), or practice different religions. As of this writing, a twenty-four-hour news cycle floods our minds with stigmatizing rhetoric and propaganda against such groups as Muslims, African Americans, Mexicans, and others.

Throughout the world, people of faith are characteristically considered the most accepting people in their societies. The very essence of faith is based on holy ancient scriptures from the Bible, Quran, Torah, and others. For example, in Christianity, followers are compelled by Christ to "Come unto me, all who are weary and burdened, and I will give you rest" (Matthew 11:28, New International Version). The word "all" in this passage is all-inclusive and doesn't exclude anyone. Even though this is a simple, straightforward decree calling all those who are suffering from any ailment or circumstance to come to the church for comfort, there are many Christians who perpetuate strong stigmas when it comes to such issues as disease, sexual preference, or poverty.

The United States has always presented itself as a Christian nation. However, the actions of both our past and present run contrary to actual biblical principles. Instead of being a shining beacon set on a hill for all to see and come to for "life, liberty and the pursuit of happiness," the nation has actually become an Empire of Shackles that seeks to impede, detain, and prevent such goals, especially when it comes to communities of color. Moreover, quite often, leaders of faith and their followers skirt responsibility by declaring that those who are faced with illness or great suffering are being punished by God. Somehow, they justify their proclamations that selected individuals have become "marked" by God as unworthy or lacking faith. Such people sink in the quagmire of condemnation and shame by further contending that God does not love such stigmatized people. Instead of offering love, acceptance, and assistance as their faith bids them, they decree a bogus wrath of God upon others who are facing difficult challenges.

Some say we are "falling away from God," but historical and present behavior reveal that we have never really embraced such a faith fully and honorably — at least not for any length of time.

CHAPTER 3

The Process of Stigmatization

Stigma is a real problem that permeates practically every area of society; it can have devastating effects and lead to some very serious problems. Our society today is fragmenting at a rapid rate under the burdens of stigma even though we have launched into the twenty-first century, where progressive tolerance and acceptance should be pulling us all closer together. The degree of fragmentation is reaching a toxic level: if something is not done to aggressively deal with it and bring it under control, we could see the very fabric of our nation, as well as communities across the globe, ripped into chaotic violence, social degradation, and economic collapse.

However, before we address the effects of stigma, we must first examine where the process begins and understand how it continues to grow and flourish in our society. Only when we can properly identify the roots of the stigma tree can we effectively lay an axe to them and eliminate stigma's venomous fruits in our lives and the lives of those around us.

The Foundation of Stigma

As with most deeply ingrained habits, stigma begins in childhood. When we are at this impressionable stage of life, our parents, teachers, social authorities, and media outlets drive into us the habit of labeling people based on a wide variety of conceived (and often misconceived) strengths and weaknesses. Parents might tell their children that they are going to be great successes or that they are spoiled brats. In thinking they are keeping their children safe, parents will point out certain individuals, classes, or groups of people for their children to avoid. Children also pick up stigmatic labels from parents who argue or talk with family, friends, and others according to how they feel or what they think about certain types of people. Those thoughts, ideas, and feelings are conveyed, often unknowingly, onto the tender, clean slates of the growing, developing minds of children.

When children reach school age, their limited view of the world has often been shaped by their parents and the environment around them. Once they are shipped off to learning institutions to acquire an education, however, they often learn far more than the mere data of select subjects like reading, writing, and arithmetic. They are also inundated with labeling training by their teachers and peers. Teachers often place stigmas on students by labeling them lazy, bright, stupid, a troublemaker, or a rebel. Students take the stigmas they have learned at home, combine them with the labels they hear from their teachers and friends, and continue the process by applying the labels to those around them. Often, teachers become witches, hags, or drill sergeants, while fellow students are labeled cool, nerds, jocks, brains, fags, losers, and teachers' pets. In today's culture, a teacher's pet is known as a teacher's bitch! Often these labels are placed upon an already established grid of misconceived views of a person's religion, race, disability, career title, economic status, and zip code.

As children are launched into society, they are exposed to further stigma-crafting by authorities in various circles. Dogmatic, religious people tell children to avoid those who are not of their faith because they are sinners, corrupt, evil, or lost, and the nonreligious dogmatic groups do the same, encouraging children to avoid the religious because they are eccentric, brainwashed, fanatics, members of cults, and so on. The police and political officials warn children to avoid certain people because they are criminals, drug users or dealers, sexual predators, or other shady types. Television, movies, radio, magazines, books, and other types of media are filled with examples and projections of stigma, which are suffused into the minds and hearts of our children throughout their formative years.

The stigma, fear, and shame that comes from being an ex-offender in the United States can never be fully understood unless you have witnessed firsthand the daily realities of being one of the ten thousand ex-prisoners, according to the Department of Justice, released weekly from state and federal prisons. Reentry programs have become a common community service for many faith-based groups and others, as more than "650,000 ex-offenders are released from prison every year."[1] According to a report in the *Economist*, "America locks up too many people for too many things."[2]

For the thousands of young people entering the juvenile justice system at an early age, the consequences of an altered life course can be lethal. A very dear friend, Sammy, who I affectionately call my nephew, grew up sailing boats while spending his summers with his grandmother on Cape Cod in Massachusetts and running through the ever-mounting snow during the cold, blistering Boston winters. Sammy's grandmother and I are very close, so I watched this very handsome, biracial young man grow up, nestled in the safety between his affluent African American dad's and grandmother's homes. Sammy was compelled to move to Phoenix, Arizona, to spend his teen years with his Mexican mother. Without the overprotective eye of his paternal grandmother, Sammy's immature, adolescent decisions resulted in a swinging door of visits to juvenile detentions. At the age of fifteen, Sammy and a twenty-two-year-old woman, after a few hours of a talk, agreed to consensual sex. Although she lived close by in the same apartment complex, he never saw this woman again. This short-lived orgasm would completely alter Sammy's life's projection. Upon turning twenty-one, Sammy was charged with sexual assault by the now twenty-eight-year-old woman. At the recommendation of his public defender, Sammy took a plea bargain instead of the feared fifteen-year sentence that his public defender convinced him would be the outcome of a trial. Sammy was wrongfully sent to prison for five years for sexual assaulting a twenty-two-year-old when he was fifteen. Worse, Sammy was erroneous labeled a "sex offender." While in prison, Sammy's grandmother moved to Phoenix to be close to the prison that housed her beloved Sammy and to support him in every way. Sammy is now out of prison and living with his grandmother in Phoenix until he can get on his feet. Needless to say, his grandmother's high-income neighbors are constantly inquiring about the presence of her "suspicious-looking" grandson. Now twenty-six, Sammy is unable to spend time with his son, who was born within the first year of his prison sentence. Arizona's laws prohibit sex offenders from being around any children, including their own. With his personality and intellectual abilities, Sammy is employable and is often hired on the spot. However, currently he is unemployed because of common, corporate rules regarding him being a felon or because his parole officer often demands that he quit. Recently, his parole officer demanded that he quit his job delivering pizza because as a sex offender (according to his record) he might come in contact with children. While speaking to Sammy on the phone, I can feel the intensity of his shame and fear through our cyber connection. Not only is he faced with stone-cold, institutional barriers to successfully reentering society, he is mentally tormented by the brutality he endured while locked up with real sex offenders and hardcore criminals. Whispering to me through his tears, he says, "Auntie, I really still can't talk about all the things that happened to me while I was in there." Even with 100 percent family support, Sammy feels trapped — and he is! A huge mistake one night at fifteen years of age is now haunting this young man for perhaps the rest of his life. STIGMA-FELON can be one and the same for so many persons leaving the walls of prison. For those of us who love Sammy, we feel the stigma and his shame.

Of course, certain labels may indeed fit the bill and be factual. Sometimes, labels can even be positive in nature. For example, parents who warn their children to stay away from a kid because he or she is a bully, teachers who warn against gang members or drug dealers, law enforcers who warn against talking to strangers in certain areas to protect kids from harm — these are all beneficial. It is when those labels reach beyond individual cases, with the purpose of protection, to include whole groups of people under one judgmental umbrella that stigma develops and becomes a life-altering issue — both for those who stigmatize and those who are on the receiving end of stigma's ugly effects.

Although we know that it is misguided to automatically label all kids who wear glasses, dress neatly, and carry pens in their shirt pockets as nerds, we tend to do it anyway. We do the same when we label all religious people as crazy fanatics or nonreligious people as devil worshippers, or apply the stigma of all blacks being thieves, all Hispanics being gang-bangers, all Asians being reclusive, or all whites being racists. If we know it is an error and unacceptable to place certain stigmas on entire groups or classes of people, then why do we tend to do it with such frequency and without question?

In-Group/Out-Group Dynamics

As we have seen, the process of stigmatizing generalizes entire groups of people who are allowed little to no variation in individual or social differences. Parents, teachers, peers, government and law officials, the media, and all other segments of society pass on these stereotypes to children and reinforce them in adults. One of the accepted theories for this type of mental processing is that our brains are designed to categorize large amounts of information into workable portions. Humans are extremely diverse and multidimensional and possess a full spectrum of complexities. However, the brain tends to place large swaths of data into more organized and compact files to deal with it more quickly and efficiently. The challenge is that we are habitual creatures by nature, and once we sort everyone into our acceptable and tidy categories, we often avoid any changes based on information that is new or unexpected. Even though the well-dressed, slightly feminine man next door is married and has children, we still categorize him as being gay, for example.

Psychologists go a step further and label this human behavioral need to create stigmatic divisions as *in-group/ out-group dynamics*. These experts say humans have an innate need to feel they play a special and accepted role in a group or groups. This dynamic consists in groups of various size, ranging from large groups, such as races, classes, and family clans, to smaller groups consisting of gangs, sports teams, cool folks, smart folks, pretty folks, and other types of cliques. When we are accepted by others in a group and become actively associated with it, we feel good, safe, and valuable. However, we tend to disassociate or stigmatize other groups as "those people."

Not only does being included in a group make us feel good and boost our self-esteem, but it also edifies us when we degrade those who are outside our specific group. Placing stigmas on outsiders makes us feel worthier, and this in turn makes them appear of lesser value than us — at least in our own minds. In this way, we socially categorize and stigmatize others outside our group or groups, often through a prejudiced attitude, which creates an "us" versus "them" mentality. Nearly everyone in our life is conveniently classified based on this in-group/out-group rationale.

The Halo Effect

We normally don't think much about the habit of labeling people and placing them generically into organized groups. It is simply convenient, reducing any need to get to know others, assess them as individuals, and learn a few of the personal details that contribute to their character. Therefore, we slap a label on them and move on.

Sociologists have found that once someone has been labeled a certain way, whether the label is considered good or bad, they tend to remain under the effects of that label, which becomes very difficult to peel off. The label remains with them and psychologically shapes them into its image. Psychologists call this phenomenon the *halo effect*. When someone is labeled a loser in school, for example, they can develop a loser attitude that sticks with them throughout life, making it extremely difficult to overcome obstacles and achieve success. Even labels we attribute as good ones can ultimately have negative consequences because people tend to strive for the outcome of positive labels. For example, it may be acceptable and even welcome for a child to be labeled throughout school as the "most likely to succeed." However, if that child ends up with an unimpressive job and attains no noteworthy achievements as an adult, the stigma of being expected to succeed can perhaps lead to depression, drug use, violence, or other forms of disruptive behavior — because that person couldn't live up to the label placed on them as a child.

It is extremely easy and convenient to apply labels to the various people we encounter in life. However, we must learn to both recognize and value individual characteristics as well as understand the dangers involved in placing undeserved labels on people. We often produce unnecessary harm for people by being careless with our labeling, which creates stigmas that are difficult or impossible for those affected to escape.

What kind of damage can stigma cause? This is addressed thoroughly in the following chapter.

CHAPTER 4

The Outcome of Stigma: Stereotypes and Prejudices

The progression of human knowledge and understanding is responsible for discovering many truths and disproving many myths associated with a variety of life situations. The effects of stigma and other negative attributes are among those findings. On the myth side of the equation, it appears that the often-quoted idiom "Sticks and stones may break my bones, but words will never hurt me" is not scientifically sound.

One recent study, conducted by Harvard University and published by the *Boston Medical Journal* in January 2016, shows that negative psychological factors associated with anxiety, depression, and hostility directly affect a person's physical and mental health on a molecular level.

It was found that negative psychological factors disrupt the adhesion and coagulation of molecules on an intercellular level, which, in turn, affects DNA methylation performance. DNA methylation is a process used by the body to develop normal functions, which include repetitive element repression, genomic imprinting, carcinogenesis, X-chromosome inactivation, and aging. When the process of normal DNA methylation is hindered or disrupted, it causes chronic immune and inflammatory-related endothelial dysfunction, which results in negative physical- and mental-health conditions, including the target issue of the study: coronary heart disease (CHD). Basically, what this and other studies show is that when stereotyping, prejudice, and discrimination are practiced, the objects of those attacks are both mentally and physically harmed. Thus, stigma, discrimination, prejudice, and other forms of nonphysical contact are extremely harmful to human beings. The data provides strong, scientifically supported evidence that high rates of health disparities among blacks, Native Americans, and other populations of people around the world who are subject to systematic racism and abuse are directly related to the prolonged and continuous bombardment of stigma and other negative physical and mental conditions.

Enacted Stigma

Joan E. Sussman, an associate professor in the Department of Communicative Disorders and Sciences at the University of Buffalo (retired), has defined stigma as an adverse reaction to the perception of a negatively evaluated difference.[1] When perceived differences — i.e., stigmas, discriminations, prejudices, and so on — interfere with the target person's ability to function fully or properly in any facet of society, it is known as *enacted stigma*. Individuals who are targeted by stigmatization, therefore, go through a complex process that sparks negative emotional, social, economic, and other types of reactions.

Most people are under the notion that stigma applies only to the disabled, mentally ill or challenged, poor, or ethnically diverse. However, stigma is found in association with a wide range of human differences, including gender, age, sexual orientation, religion, education, body type, and even political affiliation. Persons who experience stigmatic labeling most often cannot press past the experience or brush it off, especially when it occurs time and time again. Consistent, negative, projected images progressively begin to affect their lives in profound ways.

Enacted stigma adversely affects individuals who carry its weight. When entire populations — family, friends, and all other associates — are subject to the same continued extreme conditions of stigma and systemic abuse, the effect can propel deteriorating circumstances, which may disrupt the lives of many. At the same time, enacted stigma can also propel persons to strive to break through the negative images projected on them and become committed to succeeding beyond negative expectations.

Growing up in the segregated South, I lived amidst a world of white privilege and white supremacy. I grew up under Jim Crow laws in South Carolina. Our elementary schoolbooks were dirty, torn, and missing pages after being used by children at the white school and then passed down to us. After being discarded, their old books became our new books. I vividly remember the feeling of frustration when we opened our new books laced with filth and missing pages. However, our teachers, through their love and anger, pushed our young minds past the humiliation of getting dirty hand-me-down books to a vision of who we were — strong, proud black children — and who we could become if we learned how to read and write and to push past the daily regime of stigma that engulfed us.

As a child sitting in the doctor's office in broken chairs in the colored people's waiting area or being served at the back of the Dairy Queen so we wouldn't be seen, I wondered why white people were different and treated me so badly. What had I done to them? As the AIDS epidemic became a worldwide pandemic during my young adult years, I related to the emotional burden of stigma, which taunted persons living with HIV. I questioned how a disease could cause peoples' homes to be destroyed, or how children could be expelled from school, or how mothers and fathers could be driven to divorce their children, or how medical facilities could refuse care to the sick. I learned that the effect of stigma on persons living with HIV was not any different from growing up in the segregated South. Bottom line: hate is hate! Stigma kills!

The Effects of Stigma

It is one thing to establish that the stress, anxiety, fear, depression, and other ill effects caused by various types of stigma can produce changes on a molecular level, but it is another thing to expose how those qualities affect people where they live — in their homes, schools, jobs, and social circles. When we look at stigma's effects, we see that they are very real and actually touch us all throughout our intertwined lives.

LEARNING AND STIGMA

Stigma has a noticeable impact on educational achievement. We touched briefly on the effects that stigma has on children in their homes, schools, and communities in the last chapter, but it is worth looking at its results on the actual learning process. Of course, barriers in learning caused by stigma are not confined to the very young, but also affect those pursuing higher education in universities or desiring to increase knowledge through extracurricular or career-based training.

Stigma can be greatly distractive and often causes students to turn their attention to the problems of discrimination instead of focusing on their studies. Stigmatization and stereotyping are social norms in most public schools in America, especially for minority students, LGBT students, and the disabled. The result is often poor academic performance, which often leads to dropping out. For the sake of a good argument, stigmatization and stereotyping are not confined to public schools. Private and public schools alike are battlegrounds for stigmatization and stereotyping of young minds and hearts. Regardless of ethnicity, when a student is labeled as stupid because he or she has a known or unknown learning disability — or for any other reason — the results of that specific stigma might prevent them from pressing past that difficulty and reaching for greater rewards from their learning environment. Perhaps the learned behavior of "feeling stupid" is retained for their entire life or a significant portion of it, until, perhaps, they learn to apply their skills differently or seek professional help in overcoming their learning disability.

In the United States today, our education system is laced with teachers and professionals who label far too many students as stupid or bad — students who happen to be members of minority populations such as the disabled, LGBT, the homeless, or those who come from poor backgrounds. Moreover, having to walk through a metal detector to enter the school building or being frisked by a cop in the lunch cafeteria are examples of the progressive perpetuation of the learning curves of stigma upon the next generation of American children. The stigma that is tattooed on them is often worn throughout their lives. Unfortunately, too many students in this environment often become dropouts and/or inmates, which perpetuates the myth that these students deserve nothing better.

Of course, stigmatization often produces and magnifies bad habits and behaviors like timidity, hatred, rebellion, shame, unworthiness, and other types of destructive characteristics and phobias. Any one of these can have detrimental effects on the learning capacity of those affected, and, oftentimes, multiple negative characteristics are produced, which compounds the problems. As we are seeing in our communities today, too many children who are stigmatized develop behavioral problems or turn to drugs or alcohol, skip school, run away, or commit suicide.

Even smart and talented kids of all backgrounds and ethnicities have to deal with the stress and pressure of stigma. Children who are academically advanced are frequently labeled as nerds, brainy, gifted, special, and the like. And remember, although these labels may be considered "good," they sometimes can cause performance and developmental issues in those stigmatized as such. Why? Because of the in-group/out-group dynamic we discussed in the previous chapter. Kids who apply themselves academically and are stigmatized accordingly by their parents, teachers, communities, and peers often experience various degrees of pressure, stress, and anxiety, which, we have seen, can result in adverse mental and physical manifestations. Most of us have witnessed the stigmatization of, or have been ourselves stigmatized as, nerds, gifted, and so on. We may have stopped performing in order to gain social acceptance, or we may have withdrawn and thrown ourselves into educational pursuits while developing antisocial behaviors. Certainly, we know either path can have devastating consequences on one's future.

In his recently released book, *For White Folks Who Teach in the Hood . . . and the Rest of Y'all Too,* Dr. Chris Emdin, associate professor at Columbia University's Teachers College, writes about his experience and frustration as an educator and mentor of individuals who are frankly not only white but privileged, with a heart and mind to save youth of color from the dangers of being themselves and to assimilate them into the white-dominant society. Dr. Emdin compares the current urban education models to the Carlisle Indian Industrial School, the first institution designed to "educate the Indian." According to Dr. Emdin's research, the Carlisle School employed a militarist approach to "helping" the Indians assimilate to acceptable white cultural norms. The kind-hearted teachers understood their caring mission to be one of "tame and train" the "savage beasts" and assimilate them into the ideals of white society. The term *white folks* in the title, according to Dr. Emdin, is used not only as a racial classification, but also as a word associated with power and the use thereof. Dr. Emdin is clear that he is not painting all white teachers with "power dynamics, personal histories, and cultural clashes stemming from whiteness and all it encompasses that work against young people of color in traditional urban classrooms." The professor further affirms that the title of his book, *For White Folks . . .* , includes black folks or other ethnic groups that "act white" or bring the ideals of their own assimilation to their teaching models for black and brown youth in urban classrooms.[2] In most urban schools in our nation's cities, the majority of African American and Latino youth are being taught by a majority of kind-hearted white teachers who are working hard to apply their brand of pedagogy to urban students while ignoring or devaluing the abundance of cultural treasures, worth, and intellect that are intricately entwined in the urban community's fabric. Instead, today our urban youth, like Native American children in 1879, are severely disciplined and often attend oppressive, military-style educational institutions. The findings of a study by the Association for Psychological Science confirmed that black students were more likely to be labeled as troublemakers by their teachers and treated harshly in classrooms.[3] The stigma of being labeled troubled, disadvantaged, disturbed, or academically deficient is the classroom norm for most of today's urban youth. The impact of the established, imbalanced power dynamics in the classroom, coupled with a misunderstanding and lack of respect for the cultural richness of urban communities, often lead students to be less engaged in academic settings, and headed for marginalized lifestyles. Unfortunately, for the thousands of kind-hearted white teachers who are teaching urban students, their erroneous belief systems about black and brown students are sustained from one class to the next, from one school cycle to the next, and most often change does not happen.

I was personally confronted several years ago with this phenomenon when I engaged a white guidance counselor at a high school in North Charleston, South Carolina, where one of my "adopted" children was labeled a troublemaker and disruptive. (I am and have been the village auntie or "other mother" for several young boys in my family for over forty years and counting. I had known this boy from the moment he was born, and a troublemaker and/or disruptive he was not.) In eighth grade, the guidance counselor shared with me that Demetrius would not graduate from high school. Perhaps he would get a high school certificate if he made it to twelfth grade, which according to her was doubtful. His high school record had already been updated to reflect the academic track he had been assigned — NO HIGH SCHOOL DIPLOMA! I was perplexed. How does a school counselor make such a profound decision for an individual in eighth grade? Not only had I graduated from this high school in 1972, I was among the first black students that integrated this Charleston County school in 1968–69. Now, years later, with the approval of his mother, I would remove this young black boy from my high school and financially provide a private-school education to him. Demetrius's response when I challenged him on why he wrote such a perfect essay on his private-school application but showed little interest in school was, "Nobody expects me to." I have witnessed this response from many young black boys time and time again over the years. Upon graduating from a private school in Mississippi, Demetrius's ACT scores were among the highest in the state. At thirty-six, Demetrius retired from the US Army as a staff sergeant in the Signal Corps. He is now embarking on his second career.

According to the 2010 Public School Review, my high school, R.B. Stall High School, is now 88 percent minority, with the majority being black and Hispanic.[4] Perhaps white flight, school-zone redistricting, gerrymandering, neighborhood re-construction — or all of the above or none of the above — are restoring segregation laws within school systems all over the South. Interestingly, this time around the majority of students are the grandchildren of those who once fought to integrate or keep segregated these same high school halls. The one consistent element in education for the past fifty years is the majority of white teachers and administrators who continue to control the power.

As we know, the effects of stigma on learning are not confined to the classroom. All people, and children in particular, learn from other activities, such as playtime, social gatherings, and participation in sports, clubs, and other types of hobbies or extracurricular activities. If people feel stigmatized in these settings, they tend to withdraw, misbehave, or produce other forms of behavior that are counterproductive to the healthy learning process.

It really is daunting how we learn the behaviors, responses, and adjustments to the fear of seeming different to our peers. Another one of my adopted sons, Maurice, is a gifted pianist at thirteen years old. When he was ten, he began playing in the jazz club with legendary jazz giants on Friday nights in Richmond, Virginia. A student of Beethoven, Mozart, and Bach, I often watch Maurice go out of his way not to give any hints to his peers that he plays piano. He fears that he will be tormented with laughter or abandoned by his friends, so his membership at the Richmond Academy of Music is a secret to his peers. Although he loves to wear a suit adorned with shining shoes and a pocket square, if the opportunity arises to be in the company of others without such dress, perhaps when entering a Pizza Hut or Lowes on the way home from church or a performance, he will hastily toss his jacket, shoes, shirt, or tie in hopes of not being seen in such fashionable dress. Gifted in building extraordinary Lego designs, woodworking, drawing, and music (piano plus harmonica and African drums), Maurice often hides his talent in fear of being different and feeling ashamed. Of course, with my keen eye on Maurice, I am always affirming him in every way and encouraging him to express the exceptional gifts of God within him.

Bullying is now a social epidemic and a household word in America. School-age children who experience labeling, name-calling, and other forms of stigma often demonstrate unhealthy behavior that is both of a physical and mental nature. Withdrawal, irritability, nightmares, bed-wetting, loss of appetite, and other symptoms are normal in the victim of a bully. Too often, teenagers become rebellious and turn to drugs, alcohol, and other forms of escape. Data is showing that increasing suicide rates among teenagers are linked to harsh feelings of being stigmatized.

A study out of Georgia Southern University revealed that women stigmatized as "nerds" tended to be more adversely affected in mathematical performance than were men under the same label.[5] The interesting result of the various hypotheses used was that women performed more or less the same whether stigmatized as nerds or not. However, women labeled as nerds performed noticeably poorer than their nerd-labeled male counterparts, who actually gained a stereotype boost from the stigma and outperformed both of the women groups as well as their nonlabeled male participants. The conclusion of the study suggested that women tended to be more negatively influenced by the nerd stereotype than men.

JOB PERFORMANCE AND STIGMA

Because every able-bodied and mentally stable person is expected to contribute to society through some form of job or career, it is a foundational pillar of our identities, giving us a secure state of value and acceptance. When we feel good, we generally work harder and produce more at a higher quality. However, stigma in the workplace can be detrimental to performing work-related tasks.

Most of us over the age of forty have experienced stigma from bosses, coworkers, or even others outside the workplace for one reason or the other, such as being a single mom or dad, overweight, underweight, of a different skin color, or even by the type of car we drive. For most of us, the first inclination we tend to have when we experience stigma in the workplace is to work harder to prove our worth.

However, the continuous flow of personal assaults often leads to a dip in performance and opens us up to disciplinary action, workplace accidents, and various other adverse events. If not dealt with, those feelings, stresses, anxieties, and depressions — brought on by stigma and resulting in compounding problems — can lead to more serious issues and even unemployment as the result of being fired or quitting because of behavioral, physical, or mental-health problems. Once unemployed, stigmas increase and, in turn, compound the issues that result. The stigma of being of a certain race, religion, sex, and so on is magnified by now being unemployed and labeled a slug, a leech, lazy, or some other term that increases stress and therefore affects our ability to properly perform and contribute.

ECONOMIC GROWTH AND STIGMA

There are numerous ways in which discrimination adversely affects economic stimuli. First of all, businesses lose valuable skills when they confine their recruitment practices to only select groups or types of people. There is also the task of retaining good employees who are either directly affected by discriminatory fingering or who are indirectly upset by such practices. Stigma in the workplace also creates an unhealthy atmosphere in which production is both reduced and of lower quality. Once discriminatory practices become known to the public, many consumers choose to take their business elsewhere. There is also the expense of paying steep litigation costs to defend against discriminatory lawsuits. Health and other insurance costs increase in order to treat the mental and physical outcomes of stigma, and more tax dollars must be diverted toward taking care of those victimized by it.

The United States has made considerable progress in reducing discrimination, especially in the workplace. However, it is far from being eliminated. When times are economically good, it seems that discrimination is somewhat contained. However, it appears that when the economy takes a turn for the worse, stigma and the problems arising from it are exacerbated as governments, companies, and individuals become more defensive in order to survive. Racism and sexism in the workplace seem to persist, regardless of good or bad economic times. Although women make up almost half the workforce, they make only seventy-eight cents of every dollar that a man earns. On average, women bring home less money, which allows them to do much less with their paycheck, including providing for their families and saving for retirement.

Most recently, the economic housing and banking collapse of 2008 stands as a shining example of this. In the aftermath, the United States and affected countries in Europe saw a decline in social assistance, minority equality, financial and housing fairness, and other areas that were (and still are in some cases) used as scapegoats during such downturns. Ethnic minorities, the disabled, women, and other groups normally stigmatized bear the brunt of unemployment, reduced wages and benefits, assistance unfairness, and other such practices. This is backed up by a report issued in 2012 by the Center for American Progress, which found the estimated cost to companies that lost and replaced over two million workers due to discrimination and other forms of unfair stigma was an astounding $64 billion.[6]

It isn't only the United States and the wealthier countries in Europe that have been experiencing the economic woes of stigma. Most countries are being negatively affected by it. A study conducted by the World Bank on the economic consequences of discrimination across the globe verifies this trend.[7] It reported that the Middle East and North Africa experienced income losses totaling 27 percent as a result of women being denied work opportunities. It also revealed that the act of raising the employment and entrepreneurship levels of women to equal those of their male counterparts would improve women's incomes by an average of 14 percent in Latin America and 19 percent in South Asia.

HOME LIFE AND STIGMA

Home is a place we expect to retreat to and find reprieve from the hellish troubles of this chaotic world in which we live. However, home is not always a safe haven away from stigma. The many problems and issues attributed to discrimination, prejudice, and stereotyping are often carried into the home or occur within the home, where they adversely affect family relationships. Once problems take root in the home, they are difficult to eliminate, and they often cause chaos in what's supposed to be a peaceful, restful, and joyful atmosphere.

Stigma and the problems it creates infiltrate home life on various fronts. The effects of discrimination, racism, homophobia, and all forms of stigma almost always enter the home with significant consequences. My heart bleeds when I encounter gay teenagers who are fending off their stigmatizing peers during school only to be broken and divorced by their parents because they announce themselves as homosexual.

Surely, we need to look no further than America's prison system to witness the judgment and discrimination it has on families, as in the case of Sammy, which I shared in chapter 3. It matters not whether each person in prison is guilty of the crime; all are psychologically affected. Even after they have paid the debt of their crimes, each lives under the burden of society's restrictions on a "felon." In most states, felons cannot vote, there are limited job opportunities, and the stigma of simply walking down the street as a known felon often leads to harassment. The entire household is stigmatized when one person in the home lives under the shadow of being labeled a felon.

CHAPTER 5

Stigma and Health

Stigma can have a detrimental effect on both the physical and psychological health of individuals. Problems in school, at home, at work — as well as with making payments and purchases — can wreak havoc on one's emotional state, which can easily transmute into a wide variety of health problems. There is so much information on this particular topic that I have dedicated an entire chapter to it. Further, nowhere has the impact of generational stigma been so vividly displayed as throughout the health-care system and on the psychological and sociological health of populations of people.

As we saw in the previous chapter, stigma can cause various problems in the areas of education, job performance, home life, and the economy. The end result of all these problems is that stress and even psychological distress are produced in people affected by stigma, which can eventually lead to a deterioration of their mental and physical health. As people who are continuously stigmatized fall into ill health, their quality of living can erode even further as mental and physical conditions compound individuals' ability to earn money, get satisfactory housing, acquire health care and insurance, maintain solid relationships, interact socially, and perform other normal, healthy activities.

Perhaps it might be helpful to consider the impact of institutional biases, including racism, sexism, gender identity, and socioeconomics, on our personal journeys through life.

Mental-Health Stigma

Our mental and emotional states play key roles in our overall health and our ability to live a productive and happy life. When those elements are agitated and thrown out of balance, we can experience a range of problems. Of course, not all people develop mental issues when dealing with the everyday annoyances of life. However, those who do oftentimes struggle with the added pressures of stigma on top of their mental-health issues.

Experts recognize two forms of stigma that affect those with mental disorders. The first type is *social stigma,* which consists of attitudes and behavior that are both prejudiced and discriminatory against those with mental-health issues. Stigmatization is commonly placed on the mentally ill who have serious mental issues such as substance addictions, schizophrenia, post-traumatic stress disorder (PTSD), or obsessive-compulsive disorder (OCD).

Society, however, also discriminates against those with lesser-known ailments or illnesses deemed less serious — conditions considered to be self-inflicted, such as eating disorders and substance abuse. In certain cases this is true, and at other times it is simply perceived to be true. Regardless, the outcome leads to the second type, known as *self-stigma* or *perceived stigma,* which is the internalization of shame and guilt that is the result of an individual's perceptions of the applied stigma or discrimination. This can lead people to experience deeper degrees of mental illness or reduce the effectiveness of treatment programs.

People suffering from severe forms of mental illness who are eighteen and older account for only around 6 percent of the US population. However, the issue of mental disorders is much more widespread, both in the United States and internationally. The percentage of American adults diagnosed with some type of mental disorder in any given year is approximately 26.2 percent, or 57.7 million people, based on the 2004 census.[1] That equates to roughly one in four adults with known mental-health issues — and that number easily rises when undiagnosed people are considered. Anxiety disorders, panic disorders, mood disorders, social phobias, and other mental diagnoses — although less known or recognized — still cause millions of people pain and suffering that often go undiagnosed and untreated.

According to the Centers for Disease Control and Prevention, more than one out of twenty Americans who are twelve years of age or older reported current depression (moderate or severe depressive symptoms in the past two weeks) in 2009–12. Mental disorders are a major epidemic in the United States. With the daily cycles of negative cable news spewing forth immediate images of killings, devastations, and other horrors, mental disorders have become a silent health challenge in our country. Seeking proper diagnosis at any age and then getting professional help for mental disorders is vital to recovery, especially when assistance is received in the early stages. People diagnosed with mental disorders may be provided corrective medications, counseling, information, support groups, and other valuable resources that help them gain control of out-of-control mental stresses, anxieties, and other issues. Those who pursue and receive mental-health services often fully recover and return to living normal, productive lives. Unfortunately, many adults diagnosed with a mental-health condition do not receive services. According to a 2014 survey, only 41 percent of persons with a mental-health condition received help, and of those with serious mental illness, only 62.9 percent received assistance.[2]

Stigma plays a major role in hindering the recovery process for millions of persons with mental-health illnesses. First of all, because mental illness is so radically stigmatized in our society, many people refuse to seek professional help for fear of being tagged with labels such as "crazy" or "insane." They choose to go through life haunted by their problems rather than face being ridiculed and judged as outcasts. Needless to say, this leads to deeper degradation of their mental state and, as we shall soon see, endangers their physical well-being as well. As a person declines into a worsening mental condition, she or he find it increasingly difficult to function at home, school, and work or within social circles.

Second, a person who seeks professional help and is diagnosed with a mental disorder has to deal not only with the reality of their problem, but also with the burden of discrimination and stigma with which they may now be labeled. It is much more difficult for persons with diagnosed mental disorders to find work; receive good housing; hold long-term, meaningful relationships; or gain acceptance in mainstream society. This is mainly because of the ignorance of the majority that automatically deems anyone with any type of mental disorder to be unstable and dangerous — to themselves or others. The media tends to feed this stereotype by portraying the mentally disturbed as violent criminals, villains, or horribly unstable citizens who are unable to carry out normal existences.

Thus, stigma creates a lose-lose situation for so many persons experiencing mental-health issues — they are affected either by the fear of being stigmatized or they must actually face the stigma placed on them by society after seeking help. Stereotyping only works to magnify the problem and drive individuals with mental illness into worsening states of mental torment.

How Stigma Affects Physical Health

Our physical health is tightly knit into the fabric of our mental well-being. As our mental state is agitated for long periods of time and becomes weak and unstable, it is often mirrored in some physical ailment. One simple example that I often experience regarding how the mind and emotions are connected to the physical body is when I give a speech in front of a large audience. The stress and anxiety experienced by the mere thought of giving the presentation produces an influx of gastric acid, upsetting my stomach and resulting in what we call "butterflies." If, however, you are a member of the club of persons involved in a constant flow of situations where stress and anxiety levels are elevated over a long-term period — such as being stigmatized at school, work, when shopping for groceries, or as you walk down the street on a daily basis — the overproduction of stomach acid and the feeling of butterflies can turn into heartburn, gastroesophageal reflux disease (GERD), peptic ulcers, or other health problems.

On the other hand, stress plays a beneficial role in human survival under normal conditions, triggering us to move into a flight-or-fight stance. When stress occurs, the body is flooded with hormones that cause the heart to accelerate, which raises blood pressure and provides a rapid burst of energy that is quite beneficial for fending off wild animals or fierce adversaries. In today's world, we seldom have to deal with such extreme dangers unless we're attacked by someone with a weapon or our personhood is thrust into violence. However, we continue to utilize stress to acquire the motivation to perform everyday tasks well, like landing job interviews, handling irate clients, confronting poorly performing employees, or waiting in traffic jams.

Unfortunately, sudden surges of high-level stress or prolonged stress that becomes chronic are well-documented sources of numerous types of sicknesses, ailments, and diseases. Sudden bursts of emotional stress brought on by accidents, terrorism, severe weather, and similar events can trigger such incidents as panic attacks, respiratory failure, heart attacks, or other forms of arrhythmia (erratic electrical impulses), which can lead to unconsciousness and even death. Chronic stress caused by prolonged illness, job loss, divorce, and the like can lead to sleep disorders, eating disorders, heart disease, ulcers and digestive problems, chronic pain, depression (which can lead to suicide), and other ailments.[3] One of the hormones released under stress is cortisol, which has numerous important functions, such as reducing inflammation. However, when someone is under chronic stressful conditions, the body is bombarded with a steady stream of cortisol, which desensitizes cells and produces increased inflammation. Chronic inflammation, in turn, causes damage to blood vessels and brain cells, which results in insulin resistance and possible diabetes, as well as painful joint conditions.[4]

STIGMA AND THE IMMUNE SYSTEM

Stress and psychological disorders that are often caused or intensified by stigma adversely affect the immune system. Chronic stress causes a deficiency of the immune system, resulting in the body's inability to effectively fight germs, viruses, and disease. Thus, those plagued by chronic stress find that they take longer to heal from wounds, surgeries, colds, and diseases such as cancer. A weakened immune system can also drastically affect a person's mood, leading to major changes in behavior and even schizophrenia. Depression is one of the most common responses, and it creates behavior changes such as poor eating habits, drug abuse, and sleep disorders that work to reduce white blood cell counts used to fight invading elements.[5]

STIGMA AND OBESITY

Stigma concerning the obese is another plague on society that causes additional mental and physical stress to those who are overweight. Having struggled with obesity since my childhood, I know too well that stigma is applied to individuals in a variety of ways, including name calling, ridiculing, and displaying overtly aggressive actions. Living as an obese person provides a constant target for stigma and discrimination at home, in the workplace, in church, during school, and in all public and private settings. Unlike other diseases that may be hidden under the skin, obesity is who you are and can be seen by all. Thus, employment, social events, travel, and all activities are opportunities for stigma, discrimination, and hate crimes.

As with all forms of stigma, stigma against the obese tends to magnify existing issues and create new ones. It is a myth that all overweight (or underweight) persons are always suffering from barrages of health challenges. For some, obesity is not compounded by other health issues. However, we know that obesity will eventually culminate in other significant ailments and complications if not properly addressed. In addition to stigma and discrimination directed at them by others, persons who are overweight tend to live a life of self-stigmatization. The destructive attacks of stigma and discrimination from persons on the outside, as well as those from within their own minds, can be devastating for obese persons. For some, it causes indulgence in unhealthy habits other than overeating, or it produces mental disorders such as the "nobody likes me" syndrome. Persons who are obese tend to experience greater degrees of anxiety, stress, depression, isolation, and low self-esteem.[6]

STIGMA AND HIV

Stigma associated with HIV patients presents a significant problem in the United States as well as globally. HIV-related stigma places additional burdens on those living with the disease and can produce interference with the processes of prevention and treatment, research, and caring for and supporting HIV patients. Discrimination of persons living with HIV places additional suffering and hardship on individuals affected by the virus, but it also affects family members, friends, and caregivers.[7]

Since the beginning of the AIDS epidemic in the 1980s, the fear, shame, and religious dogma that promoted an austere response to people with the disease resulted in the globalization of the AIDS stigma as a social norm. This justified the displacement of human beings living with an incurable disease from their families, places of worship, and communities. Some were beaten privately or in the public square, many were denied care and compassion, scores died alone and were denied a proper burial upon death. Unfortunately, this response to persons living with HIV remains in effect in too many families, places of worship, and cultures around the world, including in the United States. The Obama administration in 2010 lifted a twenty-two-year travel ban that prohibited persons living with HIV from entering the United States. The travel ban, imposed in 1987, restricted all immigrants living with HIV from obtaining a US tourist visa or permanent residence status unless granted a special waiver. The reality of this ban denied physicians, researchers, global HIV advocates, friends, and family members entry into the United States for more than two decades. Dr. Tom Coates, director of the UCLA Center for World Health, during an interview reiterated that the ban fueled a sense of "false security" and misunderstanding that public health and prevention programs were the primary efforts for stopping the spread of the disease.[8] The facts: acquired immunodeficiency syndrome (AIDS) is caused by the human immunodeficiency virus (HIV). The virus is spread to another person only when that person comes in contact with the body fluids of someone who has the virus — for example, blood, semen (cum), preseminal fluid (pre-cum), rectal fluids, vaginal fluids, and breast milk.

In 1981, the Centers for Disease Control published their "Morbidity and Mortality Weekly Report" and described a rare lung infection, *Pneumocystis carinii pneumonia*, discovered in five young, previously healthy gay men in Los Angeles. The world is now approaching forty years of fighting the global pandemic of AIDS. The medical advancements that have been made in understanding the virus that causes this disease are extraordinary. However, there is still *no cure*. Until there is a cure, we are rowing a boat with holes in it.

Today, we have volumes and volumes of science-based lessons regarding effective, preventive measures for AIDS. Yet, religious, political, and ideological rhetoric continues to drive stigma and discrimination toward specific groups of people: men who have sex with men, people who inject drugs, sex workers, and everyone living with HIV, including heterosexual women. Actively working in the trenches of HIV in the United States, Africa, and the Caribbean for most of those forty years, I attest that there have been several debacles of the highest order by both public-health officials and congressional and religious leaders. I will not prolong this chapter by stating all the gross acts of negligence from my viewpoint. However, there is one that bears review. Federal funding for needle-exchange programs, a scientifically proven HIV prevention strategy, had been denied for years, until December 16, 2009, when President Obama signed into law an end to this longstanding ban. The lifting of this ban allowed federal funding for needle-exchange programs, which provided more opportunities to stop the spread of HIV among injecting drug users (IDUs). How many lives might have been saved or transmissions of the virus halted if science, rather than ignorance, fear, and hate, had been embraced by legislators?

The dual stigma of drug addiction and HIV has been propelled by laws that banned access needed to prevent the disease among persons who are viewed as unfit to live. One could argue that there are those who still believe that gay men, lesbians, transgender, and queer human beings are unfit to live as well. Seventy-five countries in 2015 listed homosexuality as a crime.[9] Certainly, there are many conservatives and liberals that would add the United States to this list. Today, twelve states still uphold antisodomy laws on their books, even after the Supreme Court ruled against it in 2003.[10]

Black women and men who have sex with men have the highest rates of HIV and AIDS in the world. Sadly, the fact that one in every nineteen African American women and one in two (50 percent) of African American gay man live with HIV is a loud silence in our nation. As previously stated, the burden of stigma on all persons with HIV in the United States and around the world continues to be at an all-time high. However, the burden of stigma on men who have sex with men and live with HIV is a double-edged sword. According to the Centers for Disease Control and Prevention, gay and bisexual men age thirteen to twenty-four accounted for an estimated 92 percent of new HIV diagnoses among all men in their age group and 27 percent of new diagnoses among all gay and bisexual men in 2014. All men who have sex with men do not have the HIV virus, although they are often perceived that way.

Stigma and discrimination toward persons living with HIV have been horrific since the beginning of this global pandemic. The spiritual, emotional, and physical suffering of women and gay and bisexual men, especially those in their formative years (thirteen to twenty-nine), cannot be ignored. Behaviors of sexual violence, sexual promiscuity, homophobia, and HIV stigma are sustained through silence within the population at large. This indifference quietly supports violence and bullying against women and gay men of all ages, and the relief they often seek is through suicide and other self-destructive behaviors. Certainly, stigma has supported the spread of HIV over the past decades. Fear of being stigmatized forces people into isolation or prevents them from disclosing their HIV status to friends, loved ones, and sexual partners. As we have witnessed throughout the AIDS epidemic thus far, stigma can also prevent persons from getting employment, housing, insurance, or other benefits, as well as result in them being ostracized by family, friends, and other social circles. According to research by the International Centre for Research on Women (ICRW), the possible consequences of HIV-related stigma are loss of income and livelihood, loss of marriage and childbearing options, poor care within the health sector, withdrawal of caregiving in the home, loss of hope coupled with feelings of worthlessness, and loss of reputation.[11]

An estimated thirty-five million human beings have died of AIDS-related illnesses since the beginning of this horrendous pandemic, which is still unfolding. According to the Centers for Disease Control, there "were approximately 36.7 million people worldwide living with HIV/AIDS at the end of 2015. Of these, 1.8 million were children."[12] In the United States, one in four persons between thirteen and twenty-four are living with HIV. Today, regardless of all of this death and sickness, too many faith-based institutions across the United States — and the world, for that matter — refuse to even utter the word *sex*. They continue to condemn the use of condoms, another scientifically proven preventative measure. Stigma has proved to be more deadly than the HIV virus. Yet it is widely promoted and accepted.

Stigma and Public Health

"Of all the forms of inequality, injustice in health is the most shocking and the most inhumane." This powerful truth was spoken in 1965 by Martin Luther King at the end of the Selma to Montgomery March in Alabama.

Stigmatism is not confined to the ignorant masses of society. For centuries, the medical community has been and

is still guilty of applying stigma to patients of certain ethnicities, socioeconomic brackets, or gender, resulting in denial
of service, refusal to provide quality treatment, or stigmatizing entire families. I am often asked to assist in various
ways to encourage African Americans to participate in clinical studies or health-related programs. Most times those
making the request are research or academic professionals who are somewhat unfamiliar with African American
culture but have received funding to conduct comparative
studies on those who have been historically missing from
research studies of various types. So often, those making
the requests have a multitude of misconceptions inherited
from their ancestors that suggest that black people are just
too ignorant to understand the value of participating in a
clinical study, being in a health program, or seeking quality health care. Surely, it is clear to those who often make
the requests, although unspoken, that if they (blacks) really
understood how bad their disease state was and the burden
of their diseases on our society, they would happily engage
in their clinical studies and out-reach programs. Needless
to say, these clinical studies and programs are oftentimes
run by members of the majority population, with no representation of those they desire to reach on staff. As in education, the field of public health, including physicians, nurses,
researchers, technicians, and educators, is filled with kind-
hearted, well-intentioned health professionals who truly
care about people and the field of public health, like I do.

Strikingly, Harriet Washington, in her groundbreak-
ing best seller *Medical Apartheid,* shared a situation she

encountered that leaped off the page and connected to my realities of working in public health since I was a graduate student in the 1970s. A professor at a US medical school requested a meeting to have Dr. Washington tell her about the book she was writing. After hearing about it, the professor angrily attacked the premise of the book, stating, "It's a terrible thing that you are doing. You are going to make African Americans afraid of medical research and physicians! You cannot write this book!"[13] Thank God Dr. Washington moved forward with this brilliant account of the medical apartheid endured for centuries by African Americans.

A few quotes from Dr. Washington's book unveil the demise of consciousness when acknowledging black people as human beings. These scientists inherited this explicit hate, and it continues to be passed on from generation to generation.

"[It was] cheaper to use Niggers than cats because they were everywhere and cheap experimental animals" — from a speech delivered by neurosurgeon Harry Baily, MD, while at Tulane Medical School (1960).

"The future of the Negro lies more in the research laboratory than in the schools. When diseased, he should be registered and forced to take treatment before he offers his diseased mind and body on the altar of academic and professional education" — Public health physician Thomas Murrell (1940).

"These persons don't have any money and they're

black and they're poorly washed" — Radiation scientist Clarence Lushbaugh, MD, explaining why he chose "slum" patients as radiation subjects (1995).

"Celia's child, about four months old, died last Saturday the 12th. This is two negroes and three horses I have lost this year" — David Gavin (1855).

Dr. J. Marion Sims is recognized worldwide as the father of gynecology. As such, he was the world's leading authority on female reproductive health. In the 1840s he bought slaves in Alabama and sharpened his surgical skills by performing painful operations on the genitals of female slaves in his backyard surgical hospital. It is recorded that Sims operated on one young slave woman thirty-four times without anesthesia.[14]

The impact of this extreme hatred upon a population of people has been devastating for centuries for both the descendants of slaves and those of their masters. All have suffered and all must heal. The descendants of slave masters and others must continue to "wash clean" their inherited beliefs and erroneous thinking that black, brown, and poor people do not deserve quality health care and are, in fact, too ignorant to understand their health-care needs.

The impact of the well-known Tuskegee Syphilis Study has been and continues to be devastating for America. The study concretely established an already widespread distrust of the health and medical industries among African Americans of all backgrounds and socioeconomic statuses. For this reason, medical advancements that require the participation of large numbers of black men, women, and children seem to progress more slowly.

In 1932, the US Public Health Service began a study involving 600 black men: 399 with syphilis and 201 without.[15] The purpose of the study was to record the natural progression of the disease and to "justify" a treatment program for blacks. Researchers, employed by the US government, did not inform the men about the real purpose of the study. They also did not get their informed consent. In fact, according to the records of the US Public Health Service, the researchers told these black men they were being treated for having "bad blood."[16] Their compensation for participating in the Tuskegee study was free medical exams, free meals, and burial insurance. Forty of the men's wives became infected, and fourteen children were born with the disease.[17] In 1947, when penicillin became available for the treatment of syphilis, the researchers did not offer this cure to the men participating in the study. In October 1972, the assistant secretary of health and scientific affairs announced the end of the Tuskegee study, forty years after it began.[18] The last study participant died in January 2004. The appointed Ad Hoc Advisory Panel, upon reviewing the forty-year study, found the knowledge gained from the study was very limited compared with the overwhelming, life-threatening risks the study posed to the men and their families.[19] Unknown is the daily impact and legacy of the Tuskegee study on African Americans. The loss of lives because of fear, shame, and distrust of the healthcare system will echo for decades, perhaps for centuries.

Moreover, medical research has undoubtedly been hindered by the lack of participation of specific populations of human beings, so clearly needed in many areas of biomedical research.

It is a mystical phenomenon that under our diverse skin colors, all human beings are made up of a miraculous system of cells, tissues, and organs that function in the same way. However, our individual genetic makeup, that which makes us different, just might be the one thing that changes everything and makes the world better.

This brings us to yet another horrific medical injustice, one that, consequently, resulted in *the* most extraordinary medical breakthrough in modern history. Henrietta Lacks was a black woman, born in Roanoke, Virginia, who later moved to Tuner Station (now a part of Dundalk), Maryland. Henrietta developed a knot in her womb and went to the medical center at Johns Hopkins University in January 1951, which at the time was the only facility in her area that provided treatment for black patients. At first she was misdiagnosed with malignant epidermoid carcinoma of the cervix, which is a type of skin cancer, but in 1970 she was correctly diagnosed with adenocarcinoma, a cancerous tumor.

Henrietta's doctors admitted her to Johns Hopkins and began treatment. However, they removed two cell samples from her cervix for testing without her knowledge or the knowledge of her family. One of the tissue samples was healthy and the other turned out to be cancerous. Both samples were passed along to the hospital's cancer research lab, where Dr. George Otto Gey examined them. He found that Henrietta's cells were extremely durable, outliving the normal cell lifespan of only a few days. In his research lab and without consent, Dr. Gey multiplied the unusual cell and produced a cell line that became known as HeLa, an abbreviation of the source, Henrietta Lacks.

The HeLa line of cells began being mass produced in 1955 and became revolutionary for medical research and treatments for people of all races and ethnicities worldwide. Over time, the strain was used for polio vaccine development, which triggered movements in disease research and product development. HeLa cells have been used in cancer and AIDS research, gene mapping, toxic substance and radiation effects and treatment, and many other scientific purposes.[20] Since the beginning of HeLa cell research in the 1950s, more than twenty tons have been grown for scientific and medical purposes, with more than eleven thousand patents being produced.[21]

Henrietta Lacks died at thirty-one on October 4, 1951, while at Johns Hopkins, but her family didn't find out about HeLa cells and Dr. Gey's research until the early 1970s, after a scientist tried to gain more genetic material from family members. Once the collection of her cells was discovered, a lengthy legal battle over the ownership of genetic materials and the ethics surrounding genetic harvesting ensued without any real recognition for the Lacks family. Finally, in August of 2013, the National Institutes of Health announced that an agreement had been reached with the family giving them limited control over the HeLa DNA code (genome) that was published by German researchers in March of the same year (again without consent). Under the agreement, the Lacks family is also to receive acknowledgment in scientific papers concerning HeLa cells. The family was not/has not been awarded any financial contributions in spite of the trillions of dollars continuing to be made by health, medical, and pharmaceutical industries. The world has finally been introduced to this global hero, Henrietta Lacks. Oprah Winfrey secured the movie rights to Henrietta Lacks's story and will star as Deborah Lacks, Henrietta's youngest daughter. The HBO movie is based on the experience of Rebecca Skloot, a science writer, and Deborah Lacks, who worked for more than a decade to uncover Henrietta Lacks's story.

"To forgive is not just to be altruistic, it is the best form of self-interest." This statement was made by Archbishop Desmond Tutu, Noble Peace Prize winner and chairman of South Africa's Truth and Reconciliation Commission (TRC), created by Nelson Mandela's Government of National Unity in 1995. The continuous, inexcusable practices that provoke black people's mistrust in the health-care industry not only prevent them from seeking out health care but prove dangerous for all mankind.

It is important that we recognize some changes and some of the good that have occurred over the years. To ensure that a Tuskegee-type study does not happen again, institutional review boards (IRBs) were formed as independent ethics committees used by both the Food and Drug Administration and the Health and Human Services Administration to assure that steps are taken to protect the rights and welfare of those who agree to participate as research subjects. On July 30, 2008, the American Medical Association issued an apology for racism. Then-AMA president Dr. John C. Nelson stated, "On behalf of the American Medical

Association, I unequivocally apologize for our past behavior, including barring black physicians from our ranks for decades. We pledge to do everything in our power to right the wrongs that were done by our organization for decades to African American physicians and their families and their patients."[22] (Policies of the AMA discriminated against black doctors and patients well into the 1980s.)

These apologies are notable. However, so much more is needed to address the "right-now/real-time" discrimination against human beings that is occurring in hospitals, medical clinics and offices, hospices, and other medical facilities. The Tuskegee Syphilis Study, Henrietta Lacks's story, and many, many other accounts of blatant stigma, racism, and discrimination in health care must be confronted. What is needed in public health is truth-and-reconciliation discussions, to speak truthfully and openly about the medical atrocities done to black and brown people, including Native Americans, in the name of science. Instead of continuing to label the excluded nonparticipants as ignorant and misguided, we need national forums and discussions at the federal, state, and local community levels to understand the legacy of pain and the reasons why minorities do not participate in clinical studies. Included in these discussions at the local level should be corporations such as CVS, Walmart, and Walgreens, which provide convenient clinical services within neighborhoods. All have a role to play in these truth-and-reconciliation discussions.

The Food and Drug Administration (FDA) declared 2016 "the year of diversity in clinical trials."[23] This authorization attempts to address the underrepresented participation of racial/ethnic minorities and women in clinical studies. The FDA has acknowledged the truth that the majority of participants in clinical studies are men, which results in FDA-approved drugs that are not necessarily the most effective for women and minorities. As an example, men make up more than two-thirds of the participants in clinical tests of cardiovascular devices.

According to the FDA, African Americans make up approximately 5 percent of clinical-trial participants, while Latina and Latino Americans make up 1 percent. The participation of women of all races is also lacking in clinical studies. There is now a revelation among researchers that doing business (research) as usual is perhaps not good enough. Scientific data has revealed that all groups of people do not respond the same to different therapies. One drug is not a good drug for all populations of people. One example shows that two different classes of blood-pressure drugs work less well in African American patients, and at the same time, a drug for heart failure worked very well for African Americans but not as well in white patients. Thus, the pattern of clinical studies excluding minorities, including women and the elderly, is harmful and must stop.

The future success of breakthroughs in Alzheimer's and other diseases, cancer, and vaccines demands that we increase participation of minorities and women. It is critical to the survival of humankind that we all seek to tear down the barriers that support further distrust of individuals about entering clinical studies. The promise of a cure for cancer, Alzheimer's, HIV, and so many, many medical unknowns will be revealed when patients of all races, genders, and ages are involved in research. When science succeeds, all people benefit. Sheila L. Thorne, president and CEO of Multicultural Healthcare Marketing Group and associate clinical professor at Stony Brook University School of Social Welfare, states it very plainly and simply: "Quality, Affordable, Accessible, Culturally-Respectful, Evidence-Based Healthcare is NOT a Privilege. It's a Civil Right!"

CHAPTER 6

Levels of Intervention

As we have seen, stigma, discrimination, and prejudice affect the lives of millions (if not billions) of people worldwide across a wide spectrum of society. People who are stigmatized can develop a multitude of mental and physical challenges. Persons with existing health issues and disorders often have them exacerbated as a result of prolonged, never-ending stigma on their lives. Individuals who face stigmatization are fearful that they may be targeted and are often unable to seek valuable treatment and assistance because of the inherent nature of cultural norms that exist within our society regarding specific populations of people. Individuals who believe they are impacted by negative thinking and circumstances caused by certain stigmas and discrimination should seek counseling and assistance, if necessary.

An effective game plan needs to be implemented and enacted to make significant strides against stigma across such a wide swath of society. There are intervention goals already in place, but they need to be strengthened and even altered as social shifts occur or new data is unveiled. These methods of stigma intervention are designed to assist all those involved by reducing the number of those who stigmatize and by helping those on the receiving end of this abuse deal with any negativity they may encounter.

Intervention goals, therefore, may consist of:

- The direct reduction of stigma being applied on any and all fronts.

- The improvement of mental and/or physical health conditions by:

    Promoting healthy treatments and alternatives.

    Reducing unhealthy attitudes or practices.

- Reduction of psychological stress, which has been shown to play a consistent, negative role in poor mental- and physical-health conditions.

- Improvement of the creation and distribution of educational materials.

- Direct provision of assistance and treatment to patients of both mental- and physical-health conditions.

Intervention goals are best reached by addressing and targeting three social levels: intrapersonal, interpersonal, and structural.

Level 1: Intrapersonal Intervention

Merriam-Webster's defines *intrapersonal* as "occurring within the individual mind or self." The first step of addressing stigma over large swaths of society, therefore, is to target individual thinking, feeling, and behavior. Interventions on a personal level take a great deal of time simply because you are dealing with the sheer mass of individuals.

However, plans, policies, and procedures are both easier to implement and much more effective at producing results because efforts are directed toward one person instead of many people who may have varying criteria.

Intrapersonal intervention should be directed at the two main groups of people involved in stigma. One group consists of those people who stigmatize other people or groups. Efforts should be made to reduce the desire to stigmatize others and, therefore, contain its spread and effect. The other group consists of the victims of stigma. The focus on these individuals should be to help them cope with any expressions of stigma in order to choose healthy responses of a behavioral, cognitive, and physiological nature.

GOALS OF INTRAPERSONAL INTERVENTION

Education

It is well known that it's human nature to label and even attack people or things that are not understood. A lack of understanding or knowledge creates fear, which in turn produces defensive and protective measures. Therefore, the main driving forces behind stigma are ignorance and misunderstanding, both of which occur because of a lack of knowledge about the people or things targeted. People who stigmatize others can be ignorant of various aspects of those they choose to discriminate against. In many parts of the world, including the United States, there exists a sustainable culture of ignorance and the "right to persecute" specific groups of people, which continues to be handed down through generations. The perpetual breeders of hate in our society are given the mantle of authority to discriminate, devalue, and misrepresent any understanding of cultural, religious, and social practices regarding a group or individual. Because of the hierarchal social construct of discrimination, historically, persons who are victims of stigma and discrimination because of skin color, class status, sexual orientation, chronic or infectious diseases, and so on are often seen and viewed as deserving, meek, and weak — whereas those discriminating are viewed as the all-powerful, often paying no penalty for the damage they cause others.

Since stigma and associated discrimination predominantly stem from a position of ignorance (i.e., a lack of knowledge), one of the best ways to combat it is to reach out and educate. Providing individuals with information about the conditions being stigmatized helps to correct misinformation and attitudes or beliefs that are negative and contradicting. A good example is the stigma that first came out when the AIDS epidemic arose. People falsely believed that the disease was contagious and could be contracted by simply touching the infected person or any object with which they had come in contact. Many even believed that merely breathing the air around a person living with AIDS could spread the disease. The fear and stigma that arose with such extreme beliefs spurred a massive educational campaign to inform the population that the HIV virus was passed from one person to another only through direct exchange of bodily fluids. That educational effort has lessened the mental pain and suffering of thousands of persons living with AIDS by substantially defeating the misconceptions surrounding the disease. Even after such a massive effort to educate the public, stigma and discrimination still exist regarding persons living with HIV and those perceived to possibly have it because they are gay, bisexual, transgender, addicted to drugs, or from an African country. We should always remember the disease's first inaccurate name: GRID, gay-related immune disorder.

Stigma regarding living a homosexual life continues to prevent so many of our brothers, fathers, uncles, cousins, and friends from getting tested for the HIV virus and seeking early treatment. The fear of isolation and discrimination within health-care, family, and community systems provides a sustainable wall of denial that often results in the refusal to implement common sense HIV prevention behaviors such as using a condom, having only one sexual partner, or getting screened for the virus.

Although educational campaigns that target various size groups can be offered from the local to the national level, the absorption of the provided information is accomplished on a personal and individual level. For this reason, education begins at the intrapersonal level where individuals are changed (in varying degrees) by the data they receive, consume, and utilize. As in the case of HIV and AIDS, educational interventions must be sustained. HIV-prevention knowledge is overwhelmingly unknown and misunderstood among American youth, regardless of sexual orientation. I cannot scream this fact loudly enough! We are now moving toward four decades of a global pandemic. The United States has more than 1.2 million people living with HIV, and one in eight of them don't know it. Get tested for HIV!

Perspective and Contact

Certainly the 2016 US presidential campaign that saw the election of Donald J. Trump was viewed by many as a tremendous setback in America's struggle with racism and overall human dignity. On the other hand, it was also viewed by many as an opportunity to "make America great again." For most black Americans, this slogan is a code for make America white again and bringing back segregation laws, inequality, and injustice. Stigma and discrimination among races are often experienced and viewed differently in our individual thinking, and within our collective thoughts among communities. One ideal strategy, which may be effective on an individual basis, is to appeal to a person's feelings.

I cherish my white friends because they play an important role in my life when the weight of the daily toll of racism on my mental and emotional state becomes overwhelmingly frightening and physically debilitating. Through our twenty-four-hour news cycle, African Americans, especially baby boomers, are haunted by the ever-increasing number of black men, women, and children being shot by white police officers, who usually walk free when video recordings seem to clearly show cold-blooded murder. These constant horrors of black people being shot down is a daily reminder of my childhood, when all black children knew, through the lives of Emmett Till, four little girls attending Sunday school in Birmingham, and countless other examples that white people could do whatever they wanted to do to my family members or any of my friends, including hanging us from trees.[1] Nothing would happen to them.

Too many times this past year, I have run to my white friends for a false sense of security that all white people do not want to kill black people. I am so grateful for my white friends who also desire to listen and enter truthful dialog regarding their teachings and experiences from the daily newsreels that shape their present-day emotions and feelings. Most times, we are all surprised to see the other's point of view, which is often colored by our very own stigma and discrimination. "The cop shot him because he did something wrong. He had to have done something wrong" is the response of most of my white friends. And then I respond, "Driving while black should not be a crime that results in your death by a police officer!"

Having a positive discourse with mutual respect between descendants of slaves and slave owners can be very beneficial to understanding racism and discrimination in America today. To strive for a more perfect union in America, Native Americans — who are losing their fight for their burial and sacred sites in North Dakota in 2017 — African Americans, immigrants, and white Americans must begin to intentionally organize opportunities for honest discussions of healing and restoration. It appears that continued separation from people of different backgrounds and views will only serve to foster and promote greater fear, distrust, and discomfort, which results in more solidified foundations of discriminatory beliefs.

Value Affirmation

Quite often, stigma of all kinds targets the personal qualities of individuals or groups, such as intelligence, weakness, and appearance. This often produces issues with low self-esteem, poor performance, substance abuse, depression, and other negative qualities, including suicide. Every single person has value. Unfortunately, a person is not born with an understanding of self-value. Parents, teachers, and all others involved in a child's life have an important role in teaching children self-value and self-worth. Without a strong sense of one's self-worth, self-value, and purpose, stigma can be detrimental in that it works to exact the opposite views by trying to destroy a person's worth or any value they might have of him/herself. Stigmatization actually creates a negative image in the person's mind and can eventually negatively transform his view of his value and worth. The battle inside one's mind between knowing you have value and the forced stigmatized image can be so intense that it can create mental and physical illness.

Everyone at some point in life will be a victim of stigma and discrimination of some form. Thus, parents and teachers should have a strategy for affirming each child's value. As children grow into adults, all must seek every opportunity to affirm their very own positive self-value and self-worth. Value affirmation teaches individuals to recognize their positive qualities and then focus on and strengthen them. As people learn to build images of themselves as valuable, they begin to excel in life and the effects of stigma are lessened.

Level II: Interpersonal Intervention

At the interpersonal level (i.e., between people), interventions are designed to target groups as small as two people or larger groups consisting of a few to many people. The goal of the methods used at an interpersonal level is to utilize the power of peer situations to change the entire group's behavior. Just as the ignorance or intolerance of a few can affect the many, so can the enlightening of a few affect those in their spheres of influence. Strategies for interpersonal intervention seek to bring people together under common umbrellas of understanding, respect, and unity — traits that are antistigmatic.

GOALS OF INTERPERSONAL INTERVENTION

Education

Educating groups of people is just as important as educating individuals. However, there are different outcomes that a strategy accomplishes on an interpersonal level. Informing people about cultural and social beliefs, customs, and activities assists them with seeing why they think, feel, or act certain ways, alleviating fear, misunderstanding, and the urge to stigmatize. In areas of public-health education, this strategy also helps clarify reasons for mental- and physical-health problems, treatments and forced lifestyles that stem from those issues.

Educational strategies tend to present information that disproves common stereotypes, casting persons intended to be stigmatized in a light of humanness instead of as some dangerous and unpredictable enemy. Groups or types of people that are stigmatized are also educated to see and understand the reasons why they might be considered a threat, which helps them to defuse stigmatic situations through words and actions.

Interpersonal intervention through education helps all involved, especially in areas of health. It lessens the need for people to stigmatize others, provides better environments for stigmatized individuals and groups to cope or get treatment, and instills cultural and social awareness in society. An educational strategy combined with other outreach methods can have promising effects, especially on those suffering from various ailments and disorders.

Intergroup Contact

Human contact works as well at a group level as it does at the intrapersonal level. On an individual level, the intended goal is to change a person's internal perspective, which will affect the outcome of their behavior. The same outcome is reached through intergroup contact, but at a level that affects many. A large part of the stigma problem is that people who are normally not stigmatized tend to have little or no contact with those they are often stigmatizing. This is seen so very often throughout the health-care industry. Somewhere, there must exist a bias bible that is followed by far too many professionals in health-care outlets, medical facilities, and research industries and which defines how they view black and Latino persons. Take entering emergency care as an example, or how research protocols are often established for implementation in minority communities without any representation regarding the study.

The historical and continued stigma and discrimination in health care perpetuates and keeps far too many persons who are called to provide care locked in a cycle of shadows and images, which they and the health-care system have created. Blacks, Latinos, Native Americans, and other individuals are also trapped in a state of constant anxiety, fear, anger, and other unhealthy emotions that eat away at their mental and physical states when seeking care.

However, when nonstigmatized and stigmatized groups engage in interactive exchanges in a controlled environment in the presence of therapists, counselors, and other professionals, they are given the chance to get to know one another and communicate on a human-to-human level. As individuals discuss their fears, doubts, personal problems, and mental or medical issues — among many other things — empathy can be birthed and expanded toward those whom they did not understand or who did not understand them. Once people arrive at a real understanding of those they once feared, they tend to see them in a more human and nonthreatening light. These positive qualities, which are nurtured in a controlled intergroup environment, tend to then be more openly expressed outside the group.

One of the most important areas in which intergroup contact is required is in clinical studies. As I have shared, the Food and Drug Administration proclaimed 2016 "the year of diversity in clinical trials." Diversifying clinical studies will have a tremendous impact on racism in public health. The work needed to include minorities in clinical studies requires those who have excluded minorities to open the doors of collaboration with minority researchers and colleagues in order to implement strategies that will include groups of people who have been impacted by discrimination in medical care, including clinical research.

Level III: Structural Intervention

Although there are numerous definitions for the term *structural,* we are concerned here with the form that focuses on the structural setup of overall society on an authoritative and interventive level, which includes mass media, legislative action, and organizational or governmental policies. Strategies enacted at this level are designed to decrease stigma by changing the social conditions in which it thrives. Institutional intervention within the structure of society works to decrease or eliminate obstructive barriers, encourage respect for diversity, and create a more equal level of fairness across large areas of society. Structural-level interventions can impact vast numbers of people and significantly reduce the influence of stigma at companies, education centers, government organizations, health-care facilities, and other organizations.

GOALS OF STRUCTURAL INTERVENTION

Legislation

The highest form of structural intervention lies at the top of the social ladder, where legislative methods are used to create laws and policies that punish stigma and liberate those affected. A successful example is how the Civil Rights Act — enacted by the US Congress in July 1964 — has greatly reduced discrimination in public facilities and the workplace according to race, color, sex, religion, or national origin. More recently, legislation has been passed to enable those of nontraditional sexual preferences to partake in civil marriage, adopt children, and gain health insurance and other necessities that were refused because of discrimination and stigma. Most unfortunately, these laws are constantly under attack by lawmakers whose individual positions are colored by their own religious and racist views.

In 2013, the Supreme Court dismantled a core element of the Voting Rights Act of 1965, a ruling that allows states to now change their election laws without advance federal approval. The result of overturning this law can be witnessed in mostly Southern states where voter-identification laws that were once blocked and illegal are now back in effect. Redistricting maps that allow for sustainable voting "bias" blocks no longer need federal approval, and early voting restrictions have been once again applied in primarily minority neighborhoods. On June 26, 2015, the Supreme Court legalized gay marriage nationwide. This legislation will hold up over time only if individual lawmakers do not allow their personal and religiously biased views to destroy policies that give human rights and dignity to all people.

Communicate the Value of Diversity

To defeat stigma, the value of diversity needs to be communicated and understood by all. Legislation must be transformed into action in communities and neighborhoods by local people. Structural intervention applies this strategy across a wide stage by creating, distributing, and enforcing policies that reflect these values on an organizational basis. As environments are cleaned of the animosity of stigma, individuals and groups are liberated to discover, build, and apply skills on various levels and in different capacities. For example, Native Americans, Hispanics, African Americans, and women of all races, who once avoided applying for certain jobs for fear of being stigmatized and discriminated against, now approach companies offering those positions, and many excel. Note, too, though, that many continue to face racial and gender bias and are turned away.

Media Outlets

As we've seen, mass media plays a very large role in influencing people. That role can be and has been used to strengthen stigma against certain groups or types of people. For example, the media once heavily stigmatized gays, which in turn increased homophobia in the masses. Because of the harsh stigma placed on them by society, gays, lesbians, and transgender persons remained "in the closet" for decades. Over the past couple of decades, mass media has been involved in bringing awareness to gay and lesbian lifestyles by portraying them as real people with normal lives, dreams, goals, and problems, which has helped to reduce stigma and allow more people identifying as gay, lesbian, and transgender to live more openly, free from the fear of attack. However, the perpetual, innate fear, stigma, and hatred toward gay, lesbian, and transgender human beings must never be overlooked or ignored. It is yet another assault on humankind.

Mass media has created an improved venue to continue the social thread of stigma, shame, and fear. The violence on television, movie screens, and video games is having a direct effect on the nation's ability to curtail killings and destructive behaviors among adolescents and adults alike. Since mass media is such a powerful tool, which can easily change public opinion on a grand scale, it is crucial that open-minded people with agendas that seek to liberate individuals and groups from the effects of stigma guide and govern these outlets. A great deal of good can be accomplished through positive media strategies, but, on the other hand, as we witness daily, a great deal of harm can be accomplished just as easily.

A Continuous Journey

Great strides have been made in the United States toward reducing discrimination and stigma. However, there is a great deal more to be done. Vigilance must be exercised to keep the momentum moving forward, or any ground gained can be (and is being) quickly lost. For this reason, the march toward a stigma-free society in which all people are free to express their uniqueness without retaliation must be seen as a continuous journey, even in the midst of strong head winds.

How is this accomplished? By constantly improving and implementing strategies like what we have been discussing, following up on their effectiveness, adjusting them as needed, and conducting research along the way to better fine-tune the process. Evaluations and surveys should be taken at all levels to ensure the problem of stigma is being properly addressed and the strategies incorporated are working to eliminate it. Evaluations within our homes, places of worship, workplaces, and educational settings (among others) are required. When inconsistencies are discovered, adjustments need to be made as soon as possible to ensure that momentum is not lost. If programs, strategies, attitudes, and behaviors are found to be ineffective, they need to be replaced with those that work.

CHAPTER 7

Changing How We Think about Stigmatized Diseases

From my early days in the health field as a blood-gas technologist at Emory University Hospital in the 1970s, and throughout my career, I have focused much of my energy on the role of stigma in denying individuals compassionate and competent health care. People who suffer from mental disorders, physical illnesses, or infectious diseases are faced with numerous barriers because of stigma in both the health-care industry and society at large. Stigma prevents or delays disclosure of information and causes postponement or outright rejection of support, care, and treatment. Populations that are socially vulnerable are at a magnified risk of effects from applied stigma as it prevents them from seeking proper care and getting appropriate treatment. Discrimination often compounds problems, sending individuals deeper into depression and despair, which then worsens their mental and physical states.

Mental and physical illnesses require professional assistance and active understanding from those treating and supporting them daily. To achieve the goal of increasing the health of persons who are stigmatized, we must change the way health-care practitioners and the public think about mental and physical diseases. It is a worthy task since healthier citizens automatically lead to a healthier society overall.

So how can such a widespread problem as stigma be addressed? How can harmful mainstream thinking be changed to benefit those suffering from mental disorders and physical illnesses? In this chapter, I will address these questions by offering four solutions.

Drop the Labels

One of the first steps that needs to occur toward the goal of reducing stigma is how we think about those suffering from mental and physical ailments. As it stands, we often tag people with labels to place them into recognizable groups that we assume are lesser than or separate from us. Thus, people are conveniently categorized and placed in their appropriate files of "those types," which we seek to avoid or for whom we tend to express overwhelming sympathy. About thirty years ago, I decided to cut all my hair and "wear" a bald head. This was before women began to freely express such diverse, creative hairstyles. Constantly, I was cast into a group and labeled as a cancer patient. People assumed that a woman with no hair was undergoing cancer treatment and perhaps was terminally ill. This went on for many years. I had no clue why I got the looks and stares until someone asked me, "Do you have cancer?" While the question threw me completely off guard, it brought clarity to why I was being subtly treated so differently. I had no idea that my choice to wear a bald head was an example of the Samson-like strength of millions of women with cancer.

In health care, especially in emergency services, labels and terms are often imposed on those who are helpless and vulnerable to the authority of the persons providing treatment. Needless to say, the majority of persons who seek emergency services in America are poor people, who do not have primary care providers or insurance. By labeling people with terms such as "crazy," "contagious," "dangerous," or "lost," we push individuals to make decisions not to seek much-needed medical care. Devaluing individuals only justifies the shirking of our responsibility or the numbing of our guilt. The practice of devaluing people, however, only exacerbates the problem. It makes those we label feel less human, which has the effect of driving them deeper into despair, increases their stress and anxiety, and makes them mentally and/or physically sicker. Unfortunately, stigmatized individuals are not the only ones to suffer. Devaluing other human beings may make us feel safer and more superior, but it also hardens or desensitizes our own humanity. The more we rely on labeling others, the more desensitized we become to real problems surrounding us.

Among of the most detrimental environmental crises in our country's history is the Flint, Michigan water crisis. According to the US Census Bureau, Flint has a population of 98,310, with 41.6 percent of residents living below the poverty line, and a median household income of $24,679. The city is 56.6 percent African American. After an audit projected a $25 million deficit, the state of Michigan took over Flint's governance and decided to tackle the city's $9 million deficit water-supply fund.[1] Knowing that the Flint River water supply had been declared of poor quality in the past because of the presence of fecal coliform bacteria, low dissolved oxygen, plant nutrients, oil, and other toxic substances, the state of Michigan, in April 2014, switched the residents of Flint from the clean Detroit Water and Sewerage Department to the contaminated Flint River.[2] Since the Department of Environmental Quality did not treat the Flint River with anticorrosive agents, the residents of Flint have been poisoned through their water source. An alarming number of children in Flint have been exposed to lead poisoning, which causes impaired cognition, behavioral disorders, hearing problems, and delayed puberty. There are no treatments yet available for adults and children for the adverse health effects of lead poisoning, which can affect the heart, kidney, and nerves. Lead poisoning in pregnant women can lead to reduced fetal growth.[3] To worsen this horrible story, the residents of Flint are paying one of the highest water bills in the country. In 2016, the US Congress actually denied aid to Flint's children suffering from lead poisoning. This denial from the Republican-led Congress came while the water crisis was (and continues to be) unfolding, as well as with the knowledge that Michigan officials had neglected and disrespected the people that they were charged to serve and protect. These state officials had, in fact, caused a flat-out, slow mass killing of children and adults that will expand for years.

Can you imagine the residents of Scarsdale, New York, West University Place, Texas, Winnetka, Illinois, or any zip code of the wealthy being poisoned by their state government with no repercussions or interventions by the US Congress? In the case of the citizens of Flint, Michigan, simply labeling them "poor" justifies the application of massive stigma, discrimination, and criminalization of human beings.

The result of desensitization is that solutions are not provided and society becomes increasingly sicker and more unstable — one individual at a time. Before long, we will be surrounded by mentally and physically unhealthy people who drain us economically and endanger us personally. Headlines from the first one hundred days of the Trump administration give a frightening vision for our future. In February 2017 alone, in a sweeping set of executive orders, the Trump administration *repealed* an Obama-era gun regulation, thus giving persons diagnosed with severe mental disorders the right to purchase and use guns.[4] Trump *repealed* Obama-era regulations regarding the Clean Water Act aimed at keeping our drinking water safe, dismantled Obama-era climate policies, including lifting restrictions regarding air pollution and clean power plants, and rescinded Obama-era orders curbing climate change and regulating carbon emissions from cars.[5] All of this is happening as the Trump administration and the Republican-led Congress work overtime to repeal the Obama administration's Affordable Care Act, which would result in more than twenty-four million Americans becoming uninsured, according to the US Congressional Budget Office.[6]

In health care, as well as in our families and communities, we must stop focusing on a person's diagnosis and labeling them according to it. Instead, let's turn to person-centered language that looks at the individual. This form of language separates the person from the condition they are experiencing. For example, the traditional method of labeling sees someone diagnosed with schizophrenia as mentally ill or even crazy. Person-centered language, on the other hand, respects the individual and their humanity by saying they are someone with a mental-health condition or a person with schizophrenia. The villainous disease or disorder is separated from the individual traumatized by it.

It may seem that such a small adjustment in how language is phrased would not make much of a difference in how people respond. However, studies reveal that the difference is indeed substantial. For example, one study carried out by a professor of educational studies at Ohio State University and one of his graduate students highlights the change in thinking between traditional and person-centered behavior. Participants, totaling more than seven hundred adults, undergraduate students, and counselors, were provided Community Attitudes Toward the Mentally Ill (CAMI) questionnaires to fill out. Half the participants were given questionnaires with traditional language, such as "the mentally ill," while the other half received questionnaires with person-centered language, such as "a person with mental illness." The results were that those participants who were exposed to person-centered language were more tolerant and understanding of those diagnosed with mental-health issues.[7]

Increase Awareness: Lessen Fear

As we have seen, labeling and stigmatizing people creates stress, anxiety, anger, and other negative emotions that directly affect their mental and physical states. These, in turn, can deteriorate their quality of life. Most unfortunately, we know that it is human nature to apply labels to those people or things we do not understand. Misunderstanding and ignorance are the main pillars of fear, which is the main driver of stigma, discrimination, and prejudice. Therefore, we can reason that eliminating or, at the very least, reducing fear will also lessen the desire to stigmatize, and this will perhaps lead to healthier individuals and a healthier society overall. So, how might we lessen fear and its detrimental effects?

Since ignorance and misunderstanding are the foundational pillars of fear in our society, with its cultural and individual bias attacks, perhaps we can weaken fear by removing those two supportive qualities. Ignorance and misunderstanding are best eliminated by educating and raising awareness among those who do not understand and desire to listen and change their behavior. Among reasonable people, negative and even untruthful beliefs can be effectively countered with information about feared individuals or circumstances. Then, the negative aspects of fear — labeling, unfair treatment, hatred, violence, and so on — which are born out of ignorance and misunderstanding, are replaced with enlightenment, understanding, and even compassion. However, we witness every day that people live in our world who are born into cultures of hate. No reasoning, except perhaps psychological interventions, can change the minds of those bred to hate certain people from birth. When an individual is able to attach a bomb to themselves in order to destroy hundreds of innocent people because of their religious views, race, or sexual identity, he or she has been bred like an animal to attack and kill.

Methods for raising awareness that address the issues of stigma, discrimination, and prejudice are numerous. The distribution of information can be accomplished on a personal level through one-to-one contact or at key locations, such as clinics, hospitals, company human-resource offices, schools, places of worship, universities, and public libraries. Mass exposure can best be accomplished through large, organized events or various media outlets. Strategies combining personal contact with sweeping campaigns are most effective at reaching the largest number of people. As positive awareness is consistently raised in families and among friends, or with work colleagues and within other circles, peer pressure may begin to have a positive effect against stigma instead of encouraging or silently affirming the practice, and that is the overall goal.

Build Empathy

Learning to use person-centered language and increasing our awareness of the struggles and challenges facing people we may not understand helps us to build empathy for such individuals and groups. The very definition provided by Merriam-Webster states that empathy is "the action of understanding, being aware of, being sensitive to, and vicariously experiencing the feelings, thoughts, and experience of another."[8] It is this understanding, awareness, and sensitivity to others that creates and upholds tolerance for people and things we may not understand nor particularly care to understand. Empathy is therefore an adhesive of social solidification. It is a critical element required to keep people and groups of all backgrounds and circumstances fluently flowing together in relative peace, harmony, and mutual growth. Stigmatizing, discriminating, and belittling others tears gaping holes in the fabric of social unity.

The burden of providing medical care to all Americans, regardless of their housing status (homelessness), including orphaned children or sick people with all types of illnesses, weighs tremendously on all taxpayers and on the entire health-care industry. Individuals will and do get sick, and they will require medical attention at some point in their lives. The Affordable Care Act, even with its recognizable gaps and flaws, attempts to fix our health and insurance industries that too often refuse to provide medical coverage to millions of persons with preconditions, as well as to those who cannot afford the cost of being sick. It is critical that lawmakers, along with insurance and health-care leaders, work together to find solutions to the horrific cost of health care, which results in the death of so many people every day in our nation. The sick, ill, and diseased are a group of people who are so often unconsciously stigmatized throughout our society. They are stigmatized based on a diagnosis or on their inability to pay.

A study by University of Milano-Bicocca researchers reveals the importance of empathy as it relates to race. During the study, the entire participant group (which was all white) was shown video clips of needles penetrating the skin of people with white skin and those with black skin. Reactions of the participants were measured via brain-pain matrix testing. A person's pain matrix is triggered when they see someone with whom they are empathetic being harmed. The reaction causes the palms of their hands to sweat. In this experiment, when white viewers watched white-skinned people being pricked by the needle, they responded much more dramatically than when people with a darker skin color were introduced to pain. This difference in reaction to the pain of like-raced individuals compared with those of other races is known as the *racial empathy gap.*[9] According to these and similar findings, people of a certain race or group are affected more by the suffering of those they relate to than by those for which they have less or no empathy. Therefore, raising the level of empathy for all those who are systematically stigmatized, whether a victim of bullying or an entire population of human beings, creates a greater sincerity of caring for their well-being.

Encourage Active Participation

Increasing awareness and empathy for others has a limited effect if nothing is changed about how one thinks and feels. The step that accomplishes the greatest results is that of active participation in solving the problem of stigmatism. Therefore, it is paramount that individuals who are reached are also encouraged to become active in making changes in the parts of society in which they are influential. Creating spaces of diversity is a powerful tool. Actively encouraging individuals to become part of the solution by becoming part of a coalition or committee is a big step. However, even more significant is listening and incorporating the views and ideas of these individuals into solution-focused strategies.

Active participation in changing minds and reducing stigma is a two-sided coin. All of us should become more involved in making others aware of the challenges stigmatized people face. In addition, we should all find ways to support those who are systematically stigmatized. This can be accomplished by doing something as seemingly small as embracing a person who is visually handicapped or helping an abused woman seek help. Many individuals are forced to endure extremely harsh situations alone and without adequate support, especially when facing sickness. Small gestures can go a very long way toward one's recovery. Surely, greater steps can be taken in becoming more actively involved in understanding LGBT or ethnically diverse communities. Far too many communities of people have carried the harsh burdens of stigmatism for years or even generations. All of us are guilty of discriminating and stigmatizing against another person or group at some point. Thus, each of us must begin to show active support toward hastening the healing process.

Regardless of the methods used or degree to which we get involved, any step that moves toward the lessening of stigmatism's impact on our society is a step in the right direction.

CHAPTER 8

Practical Stigma Management

Stigma, regardless of where it's applied in society, presents quite a challenge to overcome. This is the result of the fact that our need to label and separate others out of fear and misunderstanding is so deeply ingrained in our psyches that it appears nearly an impossible task to completely eliminate it from every area of social interaction. Stigma indoctrination has been occurring in various forms for generations and, in some cases, for hundreds and even thousands of years — but that is not a reason to throw in the towel and give up. It must simply be approached systematically and consistently so that viable steps can be made toward managing stigma and freeing ourselves of its very harmful practices.

Stigma can most certainly be managed, and that is where the focus needs to be placed. As we more aggressively and completely learn to manage stigma, it will continue to lose its grip on society until it reaches such a weakened state that it is all but eradicated from mainstream societal influence. The only way to eliminate stigma is to educate and change the minds and actions of all 7.4 billion people on the planet. That is an extremely tall order, yet if we focus on applying practical stigma management to make changes in those areas where we do have influence, we will make positive strides toward that end goal. It will take time, but we will be making a difference in large swaths of society throughout the process. Our primary focus must begin within our families. This infested hate can be stopped if each person begins to consistently undo the bias inherited within family structures and begins a new paradigm of discussions of inclusion and respect for all. We all belong to the human race. We are all connected by our DNA.

The following are practical management steps that can be taken to reduce the application of stigma and its devastating effects on its recipients.

Expose Problems

No solutions will ever be provided and nothing will ever change if we remain silent on stigma issues. The number one step to effectively managing stigma is to talk about it and make it a public issue of conversation. Because stigmatized individuals are conveniently tucked away into groups, those doing the stigmatizing do not know or understand the problems faced by their victims. As we have seen, when people who are stigmatized share their feelings, thoughts, and problems with those labeling them, empathy can often be the result.

Although it is very difficult, talking about stigmatized issues often changes attitudes and minds on both sides. First of all, those facing stigma should express the elements that bother them. As I have stated, stigma often causes individuals to either deny they have problems to avoid being stigmatized or to delve deeper into mental- and physical-health issues that are magnified by the stresses of stigma. Secondly, persons doing the stigmatizing must work to become more aware that the things they say and do have real, detrimental effects on individuals and groups. Therefore, vocally expressing stigma issues can help bring awareness, understanding, and healing to the forefront, where it can be more readily addressed.

Press Education

We have briefly looked at education and the positive effects it has had in some areas regarding the battle against stigma. As has been established, the majority of discrimination stems from ignorance or a lack of knowledge about the people being stigmatized. Educational efforts provide facts that expose and weaken misinformation and misconceptions. For example, it was first believed that HIV was spread through casual touch or breath. However, after a vigorous educational campaign, people came to realize this was not true and that AIDS was spread only through sharing infected bodily fluids. This knowledge opened the door for millions of persons living with HIV and AIDS to seek help, receive quality treatment, and get loving, caring support from their caretakers as well as the general public. Unfortunately, stigma concerning AIDS still exists and its impact is dreadful upon the lives of many.

Unfortunately, stigma dwells and thrives in many areas of society, often devastating a person's emotional, mental, and spiritual states. To work toward reducing and effectively managing stigma, the efforts of educating the masses must press ahead via every available venue and at every social level. Education efforts toward alleviating stigmatized issues should target individuals, groups, companies, organizations, health-care systems, religious institutions, and government operations until viable solutions and results are realized.

Change Language

Stigma and its negative effects can be better managed when we learn to change our language. Individuals who perpetuate stigma perhaps can become more conscious of how they address others as they become increasingly aware of people's problems and empathize with them. By having open conversations with persons of different cultural, sexual, and religious backgrounds, or reaching out to individuals living with mental- and physical-health problems, social divides can be mended. These simple acts by all of us can make our society stronger and more prosperous and enable us to live and raise our families in peace.

Those who are often stigmatized for various reasons must work to raise their thoughts from the abyss of self-pity, poor self-esteem, shame, and fear. We must channel the negative impact of stigma experiences into a progressive energy that seeks to explain and work boldly toward getting help and overcoming fear. Seeking to raise awareness, participating in support groups, and spreading the message of stigmatized issues will create greater freedom to step out and greatly relieve stress, anxieties, and other anguishes that compound problems. This must be done continuously within our individual and corporate structures, including faith institutions.

Change Media

Media plays a major role in forming our thoughts, feelings, and opinions. The problem is that media sources tend to use stigma to sell their productions, publications, and products to the public. Although there have been numerous studies conducted over the past decades that show the damaging effects of stigma on society, the media continues to feed stigmatic views to their viewing and listening audiences.

A consistent example is how the mentally ill are portrayed in the media. Awareness of mental-health issues has increased substantially in the public recently, which should produce a decrease of stigma in society. However, stigma surrounding mental health continues to grow, largely because the media persistently characterizes people with mental-health conditions as insane and dangerous. Headlines such as "Crazed Homeless Man Kills 3" are used, or mentally disturbed television and movie characters are shown who require extreme and controversial treatments, such as ECT (electroconvulsive therapy). This continued reinforcement of the negative aspects of people suffering from mental illness creates continued roadblocks for those who need to develop self-worth and value. Those seeking help because of negative reinforcements in the media may continue to struggle at their jobs and within their family and social circles.

Many troublesome characters are often portrayed as homeless, drug addicts, and/or dark-skinned (black) individuals within the media. Children are taught bias through cartoon characters at an early age. Time and time again, the villain in a story is the one and only dark-skinned, curly haired character in the entire cast. Media sources are rife with stigma, and the main reason is that it sells better than using person-sensitive language. Stigma sells! Fear sells! As long as media companies are unchallenged and driven by sales instead of compassion for all persons, stigmatic offenses will continue. A strong message against using stigma as a means to sell products should be sent to the media. When media outlets join the movement of antistigma and discrimination, they will become just as powerful a force at defeating stigma as they have been toward perpetuating it. By creating language-sensitive headlines, compassionate stories, and open characters struggling with real stigma issues, the media can reprogram audiences toward a favorable form of thinking that helps instead of hinders.

Change Laws and Policies

A movement to change and create individual and socially supportive laws and policies is essential toward practical stigma management. As it stands, people continue to be treated harshly through discriminatory actions by those in neighborhoods, companies, health-care facilities, law enforcement, and governmental offices. There are laws in place; however, intense efforts at enforcement and the closure of gaps in prevention are required.

Unfortunately, people tend to lean toward negative behavior if not kept in check by social, religious, and governmental constraints. We see time and time again that when people believe they can get away with illegal or unethical acts, they often carry out such behavior until they are forced to stop. The creation and enforcement of policies and laws against discriminatory behavior can work to support this endeavor.

Stand Up to Stigma! Set an Example!

Finally, one of the most powerful things any of us can do to stop stigma is to become a shining example of someone who acts in the best interests of our fellow human beings. Our individual actions and efforts go a long way toward defeating stigma and helping those affected by it. With our vast social-media networks, more people are watching us on a day-to-day basis than we truly know. By setting an example of correctly treating others in all areas of our lives, including on social media, we can enforce correct behavior in the minds of our observers.

Our health-care system can have a major impact on society within all its associated industries, such as corporations, research facilities, pharmacies, and inpatient and outpatient care centers. Although antidiscrimination policies are written, active, daily person-centered interventions can revolutionize how all people are treated and included in medical treatment and research advances, which will impact all our lives tremendously. All people of faith, especially leaders, have a tremendous responsibility to uproot some of the most appalling stigma and shame that have been put upon human beings. Young women are excommunicated from their places of worship because of their pregnancy, while the father is promoted within the ranks of the community of believers. Women are denied a seat on a pew during worship because of their known HIV status. Gay men are tormented from pulpits as exceptional sinners upon whom God has rained down His gruesome wrath of HIV disease. For generations, for one reason or another, these and other egregious forms of behavior have been the perpetual hate crimes of faith institutions, locally and globally. Perhaps a few verses from the Torah, Bible, and Quran will help someone become liberated from places of pain and shame as a victim of *hate crimes of faith,* or possibly be liberated from being or becoming a *hate crime of faith abuser.*

The Torah states in its Sixth Commandment: "You Shall Not Murder." (Exodus 20:13)

The Holy Bible states: "For I am persuaded that neither death nor life, nor angels nor principalities nor powers, nor things present not things to come, nor height nor depth, nor any other created thing, shall be able to separate us from the love of God which is in Christ Jesus our Lord." (Romans 8:38–39)

The Holy Quran states [25:64]: "And the true servants of the Gracious God are those who walk on the earth humbly and when the ignorant address them, they avoid them gracefully by saying, 'Peace!'" (Chapter 28, Al-Qasas, Verse 56)

Stigma will not simply disappear by our ignoring the issue. However, if we join our efforts as a community against this destructive social disease, we can make great strides in changing the way others are perceived and treated. Our efforts will lessen the suffering and help set free and heal masses of people held in bondage by the harsh chains of stigma and discrimination.

NOTES

Introduction

1. *Merriam-Webster's Collegiate Dictionary*, 11th ed., s.v. "civilization."
2. Ibid., s.v. "primitive."
3. Ibid., s.v. "civilized."
4. Ibid., s.v. "stereotype."
5. Liana Markelova, "Corpus-Based Analysis of the Collocational Profiles of the Terms Denoting the Mentally Challenged," *Linguistik Online* (2017), https://bop.unibe.ch/linguistik-online/article/view/3647/5505.
6. "From Tonto to Tarzan: Stereotypes as Obstacles to Progress toward a More Perfect Union," Seminars and Symposia Program, Smithsonian National Museum of American Indian, February 9, 2017, https://youtu.be/4fXxkOgesoY.
7. Ibid.
8. Ibid.

Chapter 1. The Venom of Stigma

1. John A. Grigg and Peter C. Mancall, eds. *British Colonial America: People and Perspectives* (Santa Barbara, CA: ABC-CLIO, 2008), 54.
2. James A. Cox, "Bilboes, Brands, and Branks: Colonial Crimes and Punishments," *Colonial Williamsburg Journal* (Spring 2003), http://www.history.org/foundation/journal/spring03/branks.cfm.
3. *Wikipedia*, s.v. "Native Americans in the United States," last modified June 2, 2017, https://en.wikipedia.org/wiki/Native_Americans_in_the_United_States.
4. Helen Oliff, "Treaties Made, Treaties Broken," *Partnership with Native Americans*, March 3, 2011, http://blog.nativepartnership.org/treaties-made-treaties-broken/.

5. "American Indian and Alaska Native Heritage Month: November 2012," United States Census Bureau, October 25, 2012, https://www.census.gov/newsroom/releases/archives/facts_for_features_special_editions/cb12-ff22.html.

6. "Indian Country Demographics," National Congress of American Indians, accessed June 4, 2017, http://www.ncai.org/about-tribes/demographics.

7. Dylan Stableford, "What's Behind the Dakota Pipeline Protests?" *Yahoo News,* November 21, 2016, https://www.yahoo.com/news/whats-behind-the-dakota-pipeline-protests-224501143.html.

8. Jack Healy, "North Dakota Oil Pipeline Battle: Who's Fighting and Why," *New York Times*, August 26, 2016, https://www.nytimes.com/2016/11/02/us/north-dakota-oil-pipeline-battle-whos-fighting-and-why.html.

9. *Wikipedia,* s.v. "Standing Rock Indian Reservation," last modified May 23, 2017, https://en.wikipedia.org/wiki/Standing_Rock_Indian_Reservation.

10. Ibid.

11. Amy Harder and Colleen McCain Nelson, "Obama Administration Rejects Keystone XL Pipeline, Citing Climate Concerns," *Wall Street Journal*, November 6, 2015, https://www.wsj.com/articles/obama-administration-to-reject-keystone-xl-pipeline-citing-climate-concerns-1446825732.

12. Darran Simon and Eliott C. McLaughlin, "Keystone and Dakota Access Pipelines: How Did We Get Here?" CNN, January 25, 2017, http://www.cnn.com/2017/01/24/us/dapl-keystone-pipeline-environment-protesters-trump-order/.

13. Ibid.

14. Jack Healy, "Neighbors Say North Dakota Pipeline Protests Disrupt Lives and Livelihoods," *New York Times*, September 13, 2016, https://www.nytimes.com/2016/09/14/us/north-dakota-pipeline-protests.html?_r=0.

15. Ibid.

16. "Post Traumatic Slave Syndrome," Dr. Joy DeGruy: Be the Healing, accessed June 4, 2017, http://joydegruy.com/resources-2/post-traumatic-slave-syndrome/.

17. Ray Sanchez and Ed Payne, "Charleston Church Shooting: Who Is Dylann Roof?" CNN, December 16, 2016, http://edition .cnn.com/2015/06/19/us/charleston-church-shooting-suspect/.

18. Dennis C. Dickerson, "Our History," African Methodist Episcopal Church, https://www.ame-church.com/our-church/ our-history/.

19. Dick Price, "More Black Men Are in Prison Today Than Enslaved in 1850," *Dick and Sharon's LA Progressive*, last modified March 27, 2011, https://www.laprogressive.com/ black-men-prison-system/.

20. Li-Tzy Wu, George E. Woody, Chongming Yang, et al., "Racial/ Ethnic Variations in Substance-Related Disorders among Adolescents in the United States," *JAMA Psychiatry* (November 2011), http://jamanetwork.com/journals/jamapsychiatry/ fullarticle/1107330?link=xref.

21. "Tuskegee Syphilis Study," Science Museum, accessed February 27, 2017, http://www.sciencemuseum.org.uk/ broughttolife/techniques/tuskegee.

22. "Report of the Working Group of Experts on People of African Descent on Its Mission to the United States of America," United Nations General Assembly, August 18, 2016, http:// www.ushrnetwork.org/sites/ushrnetwork.org/files/ unwgepad_us_visit_final_report_9_15_16.pdf.

23. Associated Press, "New NRA Leader James Porter Has History of Controversial Rhetoric," CBS News, May 4, 2013, http://www.cbsnews.com/news/new-nra-leader-james-porter-has-history-of-controversial-rhetoric/.

Chapter 2. The Audacity of Stigma

1. Louise Ridley, "The Holocaust's Forgotten Victims: The 5 Million Non-Jewish People Killed by the Nazis," *Huffington Post*, January 27, 2015, http://www.huffingtonpost.com/2015/01/27/ holocaust-non-jewish-victims_n_6555604.html.

2. Daniel A. Gross, "The U.S. Government Turned Away Thousands of Jewish Refugees, Fearing That They Were Nazi Spies," *Smithsonian.com*, November 18, 2015, http://www .smithsonianmag.com/history/us-government-turned-away-

thousands-jewish-refugees-fearing-they-were-nazi-spies-180957324/.

3. "Pre-War Discrimination," National Asian American Telecommunications Association (2002), accessed June 4, 2017, https://caamedia.org/jainternment/ww2/prewar.html.

4. "Japanese-American Relocation," in *The Reader's Companion to American History,* edited by Eric Foner and John A. Garraty (New York: Houghton-Mifflin, 1991), http://www.history.com/topics/world-war-ii/japanese-american-relocation.

5. Steven Hill, "Why Does the US Still Have So Few Women in Office?" *The Nation*, March 7, 2014, https://www.thenation.com/article/why-does-us-still-have-so-few-women-office/.

6. Nicholas Kristof, "Hillary Clinton, Free to Speak Her Mind" *New York Times,* April 8, 2017, https://www.nytimes.com/2017/04/08/opinion/sunday/hillary-clinton-free-to-speak-her-mind.html.

7. Chris Isidore, "U.S. Women Soccer Players Charge Pay Discrimination," CNN Money, March 31, 2016, http://money.cnn.com/2016/03/31/news/companies/womens-soccer-equal-pay/.

8. "CDC Fact Sheet: Today's HIV/AIDS Epidemic," Centers for Disease Control and Prevention, October 2016, https://www.cdc.gov/nchhstp/newsroom/docs/factsheets/hiv-todaysepidemic-508.pdf.

9. Rod McCullom, "Black Women Confront HIV Stigma, Health and Funding Disparities at USCA 2011," The Black AIDs Institute, accessed June 4, 2017, https://www.blackaids.org/news-2011/1036-black-women-confront-hiv-stigma-health-and-funding-disparities-at-usca-2011.

10. "Discrimination against Women of Color," The Leadership Conference, accessed June 4, 2017, http://www.civilrights.org/publications/reports/cerd-report-falling-further-behind/discrimination-against-women.html.

11. Ibid.

Chapter 3. The Process of Stigmatization

1. "Prisoners and Prisoner Re-Entry," United States Department of Justice, accessed May 19, 2017, https://www.justice.gov/archive/fbci/progmenu_reentry.html.
2. J.F., "America's Prison Population, Who, What, Where, and Why," *The Economist*, March 14, 2014, https://www.economist.com/blogs/democracyinamerica/2014/03/.

Chapter 4. The Outcome of Stigma: Stereotypes and Prejudices

1. J.E. Sussman, "Disability, Stigma and Deviance," *Social Science and Medicine* 38, no. 1 (1994): 15–22.
2. Chris Emdin, *For White Folks Who Teach in the Hood . . . and the Rest of Y'all Too: Reality Pedagogy and Urban Education* (Boston: Beacon Press, 2017).
3. Jason A. Okonofua and Jennifer L. Eberhardt, "Two Strikes — Race and the Disciplining of Young Students," *Psychological Science* 26 (2015): 617–24.
4. "R.B. Stall High School," Public School Review, accessed March 26, 2017, https://www.publicschoolreview.com/r-b-stall-high-school-profile.
5. Jennifer Chau, "Afraid to Be a Nerd: Effects of Nerd Stereotypes on Women's Math Performance" (2014), Electronic Theses & Dissertations. 1102. http://digitalcommons.georgiasouthern.edu/etd/1102.
6. "The Costly Business of Discrimination Against LGBT Employees," Center for American Progress, March 2012, https://www.americanprogress.org/press/release/2012/03/22/15296/release-the-costly-business-of-discrimination-against-lgbt-employees/.
7. M. Gumpangkum, "World Bank: Economic Consequences of Discrimination," The Borgen Project, March 2014, http://borgenproject.org/world-bank-economic-consequences-of-discrimination/.

Chapter 5. Stigma and Health

1. "About Mental Illness," The Kim Foundation, accessed March 1, 2017, http://www.thekimfoundation.org/html/about_mental_ill/statistics.html.

2. Center for Behavioral Health Statistics and Quality. (2015). *Behavioral Health Trends in the United States: Results from the 2014 National Survey on Drug Use and Health* (HHS Publication No. SMA 15-4927, NSDUH Series H-50), http://www.samhsa.gov/data/.

3. Elizabeth Agnvall, "Stress! Don't Let It Make You Sick," *AARP*, November 2014, http://www.aarp.org/health/healthy-living/info-2014/stress-and-disease.html.

4. Ibid.

5. David Beaton, "Effects of Stress and Psychological Disorders on the Immune System," Rochester Institute of Technology (November 2003), http://www.personalityresearch.org/papers/beaton.html.

6. "Obesity, Bias, and Stigmatization," Obesity Society, accessed March 5, 2017, http://www.obesity.org/obesity/resources/facts-about-obesity/bias-stigmatization.

7. Pamela DeCarlo and Maria Ekstrand, "How Does Stigma Affect HIV Prevention and Treatment?" University of California, San Francisco, Center for AIDS Prevention Studies, October 2016, http://caps.ucsf.edu/archives/factsheets/stigma.

8. Devin Dwyer, "U.S. Ban on HIV-Positive Visitors, Immigrants Expires," ABC News, January 5, 2010, http://abcnews.go.com/Politics/united-states-ends-22-year-hiv-travel-ban/story?id=9482817.

9. Rose Troupe Buchanan, "Where Are the Most Dangerous Places to Be Gay?" *Independent*, June 30, 2015, http://www.independent.co.uk/news/world/where-is-it-illegal-to-be-homosexual-and-which-is-the-most-deadly-country-to-be-gay-10355338.html.

10. Associated Press, "12 States Still Ban Sodomy a Decade after Court Ruling," *USA Today*, April 21, 2014, https://www

.usatoday.com/story/news/nation/2014/04/21/12-states-ban-sodomy-a-decade-after-court-ruling/7981025/.

11. "Stigma, Discrimination and HIV," AVERT, last modified May 8, 2017, https://www.avert.org/professionals/hiv-social-issues/stigma-discrimination.

12. "Global HIV/AIDS Overview," AIDS.gov, last modified November 29, 2016, https://www.aids.gov/federal-resources/around-the-world/global-aids-overview/.

13. Harriet Washington, *Medical Apartheid: The Dark History of Medical Experimentation on Black Americans from Colonial Times to the Present* (New York: Penguin Random House, 2006).

14. Ibid.

15. "U.S. Public Health Service Syphilis Study at Tuskegee," Centers for Disease Control and Prevention, last modified December 8, 2016, https://www.cdc.gov/tuskegee/timeline.htm.

16. Ibid.

17. Ibid.

18. Ibid.

19. Ibid.

20. Faroque A. Khan, "The Immortal Life of Henrietta Lacks" *JIMA* 43 (2011): 93–94, doi: 10.5915/43-2-8609.

21. Denise Watson, "Cancer Cells Killed Henrietta Lacks — Then Made Her Immortal," *The Virginian-Pilot*, May 10, 2010, http://pilotonline.com/news/local/health/cancer-cells-killed-henrietta-lacks---then-made-her/article_17bd351a-f606-54fb-a499-b6a84cb3a286.html; Lisa Margonelli, "Eternal Life," *New York Times Sunday Book Review*, February 5, 2010, http://www.nytimes.com/2010/02/07/books/review/Margonelli-t.html?_r=1&pagewanted=all&.

22. Sheila Thorne, "Race, Health & Medicine: The View from the Black Diaspora," Healthy Churches 2020 Conference, accessed June 4, 2017, http://healthychurches2020conference.org/2015-conference-powerpoints/.

23. Robert M. Califf, "2016: The Year of Diversity in Clinical Trials," FDAVoice, January 27, 2016, https://blogs.fda.gov/fdavoice/index.php/2016/01/2016-the-year-of-diversity-in-clinical-trials/.

Chapter 6. Levels of Intervention

1. "The Death of Emmett Till," *This Day in History*, History.com, http://www.history.com/this-day-in-history/the-death-of-emmett-till; "Four Black Schoolgirls Killed in Birmingham," *This Day in History*, History.com, http://www.history.com/this-day-in-history/four-black-schoolgirls-killed-in-birmingham.

Chapter 7. Changing How We Think about Stigmatized Diseases

1. "Flint Water Crisis Fast Facts," CNN, April 10, 2017, http://www.cnn.com/2016/03/04/us/flint-water-crisis-fast-facts/.
2. Ibid.
3. "Effects of Lead Exposure During Pregnancy," LEAD SAFE Illinois, accessed May 19, 2017, http://www.leadsafeillinois.org/family-safety/pregnancy.asp.
4. Ali Vitali, "Trump Signs Bill Revoking Obama-Era Gun Checks for People with Mental Illnesses," NBC News, February 28, 2017, http://www.nbcnews.com/news/us-news/trump-signs-bill-revoking-obama-era-gun-checks-people-mental-n727221.
5. Timothy Cama, "Trump Moves to Kill Obama Water Rule," *The Hill*, February 28, 2017, http://thehill.com/policy/energy-environment/321610-trump-directs-epa-to-reconsider-obama-water-rule; Juliet Eilperin and Brady Dennis, "Trump Moves Decisively to Wipe Out Obama's Climate Change Record," *Washington Post*, March 28, 2017, https://www.washingtonpost.com/national/health-science/trump-moves-decisively-to-wipe-out-obamas-climate-change-record/2017/03/27/411043d4-132c-11e7-9e4f-09aa75d3ec57_story.html?utm_term=.e25a72b43e45.

6. Dan Mangan, "24 Million Would Lose Health Insurance Coverage by 2026 under GOP's Obamacare Replacement, New Estimate Says," CNBC, March 13, 2017, http://www.cnbc.com/2017/03/13/cbo-says-millions-lose-health-insurance-under-gop-obamacare-replacement.html.

7. D.H. Granello and T.A. Gibbs, "The Power of Language and Labels: 'The Mentally Ill' Versus 'People with Mental Illness,'" *Journal of Counseling and Development* 94, no. 1 (2016): 31–40, http://onlinelibrary.wiley.com/doi/10.1002/jcad.12059/abstract.

8. *Merriam-Webster's Collegiate Dictionary,* 11th ed., s.v. "empathy."

9. Matteo Forgiarini, Marcello Galluci, and Angelo Maravita, "Racism and the Empathy for Pain on Our Skin," *Frontiers in Psychology,* May 23, 2011, http://journal.frontiersin.org/article/10.3389/fpsyg.2011.00108/full.

ABOUT THE AUTHOR

Pernessa C. Seele is the founder and CEO of The Balm In Gilead, Inc., a not-for-profit organization celebrating three decades of providing technical training and services that strengthen the capacity of faith institutions in the United States and Africa to promote health education, disease management, 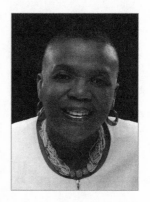 and services, which contributes to the elimination of human suffering. She was named by *Time* magazine as One of the Most Influential Persons in the World. *Essence* magazine, in its thirty-fifth anniversary issue, selected her as one of 35 Most Beautiful and Remarkable Women in the World. *Ebony* magazine named her one of its Power 150, and she was selected by *Women's E-News* as one of its twenty-one Leaders for the 21st Century. Dr. Seele is a licensed minister. She is a native of Lincolnville, South Carolina.

Berrett–Koehler
Publishers

Berrett-Koehler is an independent publisher dedicated to an ambitious mission: *Connecting people and ideas to create a world that works for all.*

We believe that the solutions to the world's problems will come from all of us, working at all levels: in our organizations, in our society, and in our own lives. Our BK Business books help people make their organizations more humane, democratic, diverse, and effective (we don't think there's any contradiction there). Our BK Currents books offer pathways to creating a more just, equitable, and sustainable society. Our BK Life books help people create positive change in their lives and align their personal practices with their aspirations for a better world.

All of our books are designed to bring people seeking positive change together around the ideas that empower them to see and shape the world in a new way.

And we strive to practice what we preach. At the core of our approach is Stewardship, a deep sense of responsibility to administer the company for the benefit of all of our stakeholder groups including authors, customers, employees, investors, service providers, and the communities and environment around us. Everything we do is built around this and our other key values of quality, partnership, inclusion, and sustainability.

This is why we are both a B-Corporation and a California Benefit Corporation—a certification and a for-profit legal status that require us to adhere to the highest standards for corporate, social, and environmental performance.

We are grateful to our readers, authors, and other friends of the company who consider themselves to be part of the BK Community. We hope that you, too, will join us in our mission.

A BK Currents Book

BK Currents books bring people together to advance social and economic justice, shared prosperity, sustainability, and new solutions for national and global issues. They advocate for systemic change and provide the ideas and tools to solve social problems at their root. So get to it!

To find out more, visit **www.bkconnection.com**.

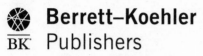

Berrett–Koehler
Publishers

Connecting people and ideas
to create a world that works for all

Dear Reader,

Thank you for picking up this book and joining our worldwide community of Berrett-Koehler readers. We share ideas that bring positive change into people's lives, organizations, and society.

To welcome you, we'd like to offer you a free e-book. You can pick from among twelve of our bestselling books by entering the promotional code **BKP92E** here: http://www.bkconnection.com/welcome.

When you claim your free e-book, we'll also send you a copy of our e-newsletter, the *BK Communiqué*. Although you're free to unsubscribe, there are many benefits to sticking around. In every issue of our newsletter you'll find

- A free e-book
- Tips from famous authors
- Discounts on spotlight titles
- Hilarious insider publishing news
- A chance to win a prize for answering a riddle

Best of all, our readers tell us, "Your newsletter is the only one I actually read." So claim your gift today, and please stay in touch!

Sincerely,

Charlotte Ashlock
Steward of the BK Website

Questions? Comments? Contact me at bkcommunity@bkpub.com.

Certified

Corporation
bcorporation.net